HYDROGEN PEROXIDE
Medical
Miracle

William Campbell Douglass, MD

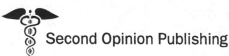

Second Opinion Publishing

Second Opinion Publishing also publishes Dr. Douglass' monthly "contrary opinion" medical newsletter, *Second Opinion*. To subscribe or obtain a free catalog describing all *Second Opinion* products, please call or write:

Second Opinion Publishing, Inc.
P.O. Box 467939
Atlanta, GA 31146-7939
1-800-728-2288 or 1-770-399-5617

Contents

Dedication

To Charles H. Farr, M.D., Ph. D.,
to whom the world owes a great debt.

Foreword

What's going on here? Peroxides are supposed to be bad for you. Free radicals and all that. But now we hear that hydrogen peroxide is *good* for us.

I have been very skeptical about this one, but so many patients were asking my opinion about H₂O₂ that it was getting embarrassing to say, "I don't know." I didn't want to give up Monday Night Football to research H₂O₂, but there was just no way out of it. (The games were lousy anyway.)

I was astounded to find that excellent clinical research had been done on the medical uses of hydrogen peroxide as far back as 1914! (There goes my Monday Night Football — maybe Sunday afternoon, too.)

Doctor J.S. Haldone reported in 1919 that oxygen dissolved in the blood would probably be a good way to combat infection. (Remember that in those days infection was it. If you didn't get stomped to death by a horse, you would most likely die of infection. Cancer was not a scourge and cardiovascular disease had not been invented yet.)

Hydrogen peroxide will put extra oxygen in your blood. There's no doubt about that. But *prevailing expert opinion is* that it has no value. The red cells must transport oxygen for effective oxygen delivery, they tell us. But this is manifestly untrue. Hyperbaric oxygen therapy, for instance, where oxygen is forced into the blood under pressure, can be lifesaving in carbon monoxide poisoning, cyanide poisoning, and smoke inhalation.

But pushing oxygen into the blood by using pressure

is an expensive business. A hyperbaric oxygen unit costs about $100,000. Hydrogen peroxide costs pennies. So if you can get oxygen into the blood cheaply and safely, maybe cancer (which doesn't like oxygen), emphysema, AIDS, and many other terrible diseases can be treated effectively.

Intravenous hydrogen peroxide rapidly relieves allergic reactions, influenza symptoms, and acute viral infections. These effects are thought to be due to the oxidation of the various foreign substances in the blood.

Tumor cells, bacteria, and other unwanted foreign elements in the blood can usually be destroyed with hydrogen peroxide treatment. Peroxide has a definite destructive effect on tumors, and, in fact, cancer therapy may prove to be the most dramatic and useful place for peroxide therapy.[1]

No one expects to live forever. But we would all like to have a George Burns finish. The prospect of finishing life in a nursing home after abandoning your tricycle in the mobile home park is not appealing. Then comes the loss of control of vital functions — the ultimate humiliation. Is life supposed to be from tricycle to tricycle and diaper to diaper? You come into this world crying, but do you have to leave crying? I don't believe you do. And you won't either after you see the evidence.

Sounds too good to be true, doesn't it? Read on and decide for yourself.

                              William Campbell Douglass, M.D.

Introduction

Hydrogen Peroxide, peroxide, and H_2O_2 are terms which will be used interchangeably throughout this book.

We are going to start with some quotes from a doctor of medicine, Peter Gott, M.D. He is passionately and irrevocably dedicated to the practice (and science) of medicine as it is defined (and enforced) by the great fountain of knowledge represented by the Mayo Clinic, Harvard, The P.N.E.J.M. (The Prestigious *New England Journal of Medicine*), and the American Medical Association (AMA).

Dr. Gott attacks viciously and acerbically anything that he perceives to be heretical, while ignoring the basic research and clinical research that has appeared in *his own revered conventional scientific literature*.

It's what I call *scientific scotomata*. Scotomata are blind spots in the visual field. On a test screen used by an eye doctor, these will be black blobs in various parts of the field of vision. There are many causes for this eye disease. The scotomata of the intellect seen in many scientists, especially medical scientists, is not a physical but an intellectual affliction.

We are taught in medical school, in subtle ways, that you can't trust any research findings that don't have the blessing of the temples of learning and bastions of the *status quo* mentioned above, *even if that research was done in a respected center by a respected researcher.* Look at the way they drove Dr. George Crile out of the Temple of Medicine for reporting, after years of careful research, that radical breast cancer surgery is a waste of time. His research was done at the Cleveland Clinic. Doctor Linus Pauling, a Nobel prize winner, got the same treatment for his work on vitamin C and cancer.

Doctor Gott writes a syndicated column in which he attacks anything in medicine that he considers to be heresy. One of his recent attacks was on hydrogen peroxide, the subject of this book. Doctor Gott has apparently, from the content of his remarks, had no experience with H_2O_2 beyond the bleaching of hair. He says that hydrogen peroxide is for external use only and especially for *women who are convinced that blondes have more fun.*

Dr. Gott *knows* that he is right because he is a doctor who *embraces scientific methods* — *like* calling peroxide therapy knavery — without having bothered to research the scientific literature. Gott is in for a surprise — if he ever does his homework.

In one of his sarcastic articles[1] he lists what I call *ha ha* items to show his contempt for some of the claims made by researchers associated with hydrogen peroxide:

Micro-organisms give off calcium waste matter that cements bones together — *ha ha.*

They lodge in liver and kidneys — *ha ha.*

And they line the arteries causing hard deposits on the arterial walls — *ha ha.*

Gott is apparently too convulsed with laughter to tell you that the basic research from which these claims were derived was done by Dr. Edward C. Rosenow, author of 450 published medical papers and an associate at the Mayo Clinic for over 60 years! *(Ha Ha).* Dr. Rosenow proved *over 80 years ago* (1914) that bacteria could be found consistently in the lymph nodes that drain joints.[2] He was probably the first scientist to postulate that H_2O_2 would help arthritis because of its ability to supply oxygen to oxygen-hating organisms causing arthritis (*streptococcus viridans*).

I have reviewed the scientific literature of the past 176 years on hydrogen peroxide; hundreds of articles on such subjects as: "Catalysis of single oxygen production in the reaction of hydrogen peroxide and hypochlorous acid by diazabicyclo octane."

Can you imagine how boring it is to wade through that kind of sanskrit to get to the good stuff? (I hope you show your appreciation by buying a lot of these books.)

Walter Grotz, one of the pioneers in oral peroxide therapy, has a keen and inquisitive mind. Although he is an ex-bureaucrat himself (retired postmaster), he understands and dislikes bureaucracy like most of the rest of us. And Mr. Grotz understands something else that many don't understand. All of the bureaucracy and self-serving bureaucrats are not in the government.

Take the American Cancer Society, for instance. Grotz took peroxide by mouth, and in 16 days his arthritis had improved dramatically. He called the American Cancer Society and asked their opinion of hydrogen peroxide therapy. The representative who answered the phone said it was quackery.

"You mean a therapy that costs a lot of money and doesn't do any good?" he asked. "Yes," she replied, "that's the best explanation I have heard. It costs a lot of money and doesn't do any good."

His treatment cost less than six dollars.

Walter Grotz discovered something else that dispels a myth about H_2O_2. Ask the average scientist if he would expect to find any oxygen left after boiling and distilling hydrogen peroxide. He would probably say no, because H_2O_2 has a boiling point of 152 degrees Fahrenheit. You don't have to heat it much to make it boil. But, surprisingly, after distilling there is still considerable oxygen left in the fluid. It's a quirk of nature. Undoubtedly, there is a scientific explanation, but I don't know what it is.

There are a number of products on the market that claim to supply oxygen to the body better and more safely than H_2O_2. These products (Aerox, Di-Oxychloride, Anti-Oxid-10, and others) are simply a very expensive method of doing what H_2O_2 will do for pennies.

A comparison of peroxide[3] with these little bottles reveals that hydrogen peroxide contains *94 percent oxygen*. The dropper bottles contain 47 percent oxygen, which comes from chlorine peroxide.

The peroxide, which is dirt cheap, breaks down into water and oxygen. The chlorine peroxide breaks down into chlorine and oxygen. So at equal volumes, you get *twice as much oxygen* from peroxide and no chlorine (which you don't need, although it does no harm in such small quantities).

So you are actually paying *$40 an ounce* for your oxygen in these products. (They cost $20 an ounce, and up, but are less than 50 percent oxygen.) Peroxide can be obtained for $.40 a pint. Take your choice.

Chapter 1

The Roots of a Remarkable Therapy

The Indians (as in India) have been fascinated by oxygen as a therapy for a long time. Back in 1940, Doctors Inderjit Singh and Mangaldas Shah of Bombay, India experimented on oxygen given intravenously.[1]

But the concept goes back even further. O_2 therapy was discussed in the *Lancet* for the first time in 1916.

Drs. Turnicliffe and Stebbing noted in their Lancet article[2] that Nysten had used O_2 successfully in dogs in France in 1811: "The animal seemed entirely unaffected by the injections" (i.e., no side effects).

They also pointed out that Doctor Demarquay, in 1886, made the observation that the oxygen given was not completely eliminated by the lungs and, therefore, went to the tissues.[3] He made this simple and very astute observation by cutting the animal and noting that the blood was bright red, rather than the usual dark red of the venous blood. This observation was recently confirmed with modern, precise instruments.

With these encouraging reports from the old French literature, Turnicliffe and Stebbing in England tried pure oxygen intravenously for the first time in humans in 1916.

Their conclusions from their experiments were unequivocal: *The intravenous method of oxygen administration, if carefully carried out ... is available to the clinician and will give therapeutic results.*

Doctors being doctors, they became victims of the "Tomato Effect." Everyone, including "scientific authorities" in the 18th century, knew that tomatoes were poisonous. So, today, "everyone knows" that hydrogen peroxide cannot be used as a therapeutic agent. If this were not so, we would have read about it in the *Journal of the American Medical Association* (*JAMA*). A quick look at a copy of the *JAMA* will tell you why doctors don't know about peroxide "bio-oxidative" therapy. Drug companies, through their advertising, foot the bill for the journal. Cheap peroxide therapy would put many of them out of business.

Our Indian friend, Doctor Singh, attempted in 1932 to give oxygen under the skin and into the abdominal cavity. He found that the amount absorbed was too small to be of practical value. The first recorded use of peroxide in this country was by a Georgia doctor located, I'm proud to say, a short walk from my former office. In 1888, Dr. P.L Cortelyou of Marietta, Georgia, reported on the use of peroxide in treatment of diseases of the nose and throat.

In one case of diphtheria, often fatal in those days, he used a nasal spray of peroxide, and the patient was well in one day.

Many other attempts at oxygen therapy were made between 1811 and 1935. But researchers lost interest with the advent of the drug era in medicine, starting around 1940.

Intravenous oxygen therapy isn't the only promising line of research that was dropped with the advent of the pharmaceutical revolution. Homeopathy, herbology, electro-medicine, and a lot of other promising lines of research were thrown out. Drugs were in. That's where the research money was (and is). Drugs were going to solve all of our medical problems.

We now know that drugs are *not* going to solve all of our problems. Some researchers are going back to basics and taking up research that never should have been dropped, like oxygen therapy.

Going back to 1940 and Dr. Singh, the last of the early pioneers of oxygen therapy, he found that dogs could be kept alive for 16 minutes on intravenous oxygen — without any air going through the lungs. It's usually curtains within three to five minutes.

He next tried giving oxygen in the vein to patients dying of pneumonia. Pneumonia was another deadly disease in those days. The antibiotics deserve some credit here for saving people from death due to pneumonia. (But they get more credit than they deserve.)

Out of six cases given the intravenous oxygen, five died. One typical report: "There was distinct clinical improvement, but the patient died after seven days."

Hmmm.

The one in six who lived wasn't as sick as the others. There was little oxygen research done for the next 20 years. I guess I would have gotten discouraged, too.

A German doctor, H.S. Regelsberger, wrote a book on the oxygenation of blood for the treatment of high blood pressure. He theorized that oxygenation would reduce the viscosity or thickness of blood and thereby reduce blood pressure. The theory proved to be correct. His book, *Oxygenation,* should be required reading for all medical students. (I've been trying to locate a copy — no luck.)

Dr. Edward Carl Rosenow's 450 published papers should also be required reading. *But they have disappeared into the memory hole.* It's the strangest thing. I looked him up in the authors index at the Emory University medical library. There were no references to any of his peroxide research. A call to the Mayo Clinic was a waste of my nickel. The girl I talked to didn't know who I was talking about.

The researchers at Baylor University had their funding cut off, although their findings were sensational. Is there a conspiracy here? Seems like it to me.

In 1920, Doctors Oliver and Cantab reported to the *Lancet* on the use of hydrogen peroxide in a series of pneumonia cases in India. An 80 percent mortality was being experienced among Indian troops from pneumonia.

Doctors Oliver and Cantab made a bold move against

this devastating epidemic. They decided to do the unthinkable — inject hydrogen peroxide directly into the vein. Textbooks warned that gas embolism, a dreaded condition causing strokes through bubbles in the brain, would result from intravenous hydrogen peroxide administration.

The doctors felt they had little to lose. The soldiers were dropping faster than in a battle with the Gurkas. They treated only those cases that were considered hopeless. Out of these they saved about 50 percent — 13 out of 25 lived. All would have died without hydrogen peroxide. There was none of the dreaded gas embolism or any other side-effects.

What was the mechanism of these remarkable recoveries from a terminal condition? You'd think that if the oxygen is stimulating the good cells, then the bugs causing the problem would also be stimulated. What apparently happens is that the toxins formed by the bacteria or virus are *oxidized* by the oxygen. (That's just my theory. I'm open to suggestions.)

They point out that hydrogen peroxide has always been assumed to be toxic to cells. Boy, were we wrong. It now appears H_2O_2 is an *essential metabolite*. That means it's not toxic, but *essential to life's process*. How's that for a switch? Doctor Rannasarma of the Indian Institute of Science says, "The generation of H_2O_2 in cellular processes seems to be purposeful and H_2O_2 cannot be dismissed as a mere undesirable by-product."

Another terrible condition that often leads to death, unless massive antibiotic therapy is combined with hyperbaric oxygen, is gas gangrene, an infection that follows severe lacerating injury or surgery.[4] The bacteria involved create a gas that invades the tissues. The tissues swell to enormous size due to the gas formation, and the most unimaginable smell emanates from the infected tissue. It's literally the smell of death, the smell of the battlefield. If untreated, the victim will die within 48 hours.

Like cancer cells, the bacteria that cause gas gangrene

thrive without oxygen, so the treatment of choice has been massive doses of penicillin combined with hyperbaric oxygen (HBO). But HBO is not readily available, and probably never will be.

Two Indian doctors in New Delhi, India, experimented on dogs given a gas gangrene infection. The dogs were injected with two billion gas-forming organisms into the muscle of a leg. One set of dogs received H_2O_2 treatment through an artery leading to the infection site. The other set of dogs got the inoculations of gas gangrene bacteria but no H_2O_2.

The dogs not getting the H_2O_2 developed the usual stinking, rotten infection with sloughing of skin and muscle. They all eventually died of septicemia. Of the 10 dogs treated with H_2O_2, only two developed gas gangrene infection.

Gas gangrene is most commonly seen under wartime conditions. If medical science would only recognize the importance of this long-neglected therapy, many battlefield tragedies could be avoided at little cost.

Chapter 2

It Really Works — But How?

Hydrogen peroxide, which properly should be called hydrogen dioxide, is a colorless (blue in thick layers), odorless liquid. Its melting point is minus two degrees Celsius, and its boiling point is 152 degrees Celsius. It is soluble in water at all concentrations and it is usually encountered as a dilute solution of three percent. Hydrogen peroxide is used (1) as a bleaching agent; (2) as an antiseptic and disinfectant; (3) as an oxidizing agent, and (4) as an oxidizer in rocket motors for small rockets.

Hydrogen peroxide solutions dismutate (i.e., break down) slowly when undisturbed at about the rate of one percent per month. Contrary to popular belief, hydrogen peroxide is not unstable, and even when heated, it will break down very slowly. If this dismutation reaction is rapidly increased in the presence of contaminants such as dust, metal, or glass, it may be quite explosive. Cold retards the dismutation and solutions may be refrigerated or stored at temperatures below zero degrees Celsius. Hydrogen peroxide occurs only in traces in nature, mostly in rain and snow. It has not yet been detected in interstellar space.[1]

Early studies on H_2O_2 infusions predicted that its half-life is less than one-tenth of a second. However, more recent studies by MacNaughton calculated that the half-life of peroxide ranges from three-quarters of a second to two seconds and is dependent upon the rate of mixing in the blood.

All species of animals do not react the same to peroxide because there are species differences in catalase enzyme content between man and animal. So the results from many animal models will not correlate with what happens in man and, therefore, are not applicable to man. Dogs and chickens, for instance, have very low catalase levels, and so they have poor tolerance to H_2O_2. In fact, you can kill them with hydrogen peroxide. They will develop pulmonary edema and methemoglobinemia. However, in man, catalase is abundant in both the plasma and red cells and is significantly elevated in diseases such as rheumatoid arthritis.[2] It can be used in dogs, as you will soon see from the reports in this chapter. You just have to be careful.

Hydrogen peroxide initially reacts with catalase in the plasma and the white blood cells. Later, it penetrates the cell membrane of erythrocytes (red blood cells), where it reacts with catalase within the cell, and additional oxygen is then released.

Some of the biological killing activities of hydrogen peroxide may be attributed to interferon. Production of interferon by human killer cells and monocytes is stimulated by hydrogen peroxide.

Studies have been done comparing hyperbaric oxygen (giving the patient oxygen under pressure in a high pressure tank) and intravenous hydrogen peroxide to compare the level of the oxygen content in tissues.[3] These researchers found that the tissue oxygen levels with intravenous hydrogen peroxide paralleled the increase in oxygen found with hyperbaric oxygen pressure treatment. This is a very important finding, because hyperbaric oxygen treatment is expensive, does have some risks, is rather cumbersome, and is generally not available.

Conversely, intravenous hydrogen peroxide is more readily available, is relatively cheap, safe, and quite effective. Also of great importance, Dr. Charles Farr found that increased oxygen content of tissues often was not recorded until 40 to 45 minutes after the beginning of the peroxide injection. This probably explains why some investigators did not find a rise in the tissue oxygen pressure, because they measured it too soon. These investigators speculated that any increased venous oxygen saturation in tissues would be lost by diffusion of oxygen in the pulmonary capillary bed of the lungs. But Farr found this to be in error.[4]

If you're not interested in the physiological reasons why Dr. Farr found previous assumptions to be in error concerning the amount of oxygen absorbed through intravenous hydrogen peroxide, we suggest you skip the following paragraph:

If oxygen, released from intravenous H_2O_2, diffuses from the pulmonary capillary bed into the alveolar space, alveolar pO_2 will rapidly increase and pulmonary capillary blood pO_2 will decrease. Diffusion into the alveoli will occur more rapidly than the alveolar loss of oxygen to respiratory exchange. Inspired oxygen added to the oxygen diffused into the alveoli from the pulmonary capillary at the arterial end would increase the alveolar pO_2 greater than the blood pO_2 at the venous end of the capillary. The increased pO_2 in the alveolus would cause the oxygen to rapidly diffuse back into the pulmonary capillary at the venous side and go back into systemic circulation. This postulate was confirmed by studies of pulmonary oxygen uptake to determine metabolic rate in subjects receiving various concentrations of intravenous hydrogen peroxide.[5]

Welcome back.

We have noted, as has Dr. Farr, that blood specimens taken during and after hydrogen peroxide infusions show a color change consistent with an increase in oxygen content of the blood after the infusion. We sent a sample to the laboratory, and, although it was a venous specimen, the lab reported back that it must have been an arterial sample because of the high oxygen color of the blood.

After an hour of infusion of hydrogen peroxide, a 2-10 percent decrease will be noted in many blood constituents — such as sodium, potassium, chloride, phosphorus, etc. Twenty-four hours later, all of these constituents of the blood will have returned to normal pre-infusion levels.

*****

The clinical benefit of oxygen saturation of tissue
fluid from the oxygen produced by hydrogen peroxide
may be of secondary importance. Very little peroxide is
used in the treatment and, hence, very little oxygen is actually produced. Hydrogen peroxide is a powerful oxidizer, however, and will oxidize toxic and nontoxic
substances alike, which is completely separate from its
role as an oxygen contributor. Farr describes the biologic
effects observed from the intravenous administration of
H_2O_2 as "oxidative detoxification." The oxidative benefits
may include the oxidation of lipid material in the vessel
wall to reverse atherosclerosis.[6] There are many other
physiological benefits to *oxidative detoxification*, but it is too
technical for this book. However, if you wish to investigate
further, we recommend the article by Weiss, in the *Journal
of Clinical Investigation* (1981;68:714-721). Weiss discusses
things that I'm sure you remember from your high school
biology course, such as aggregated immuno-globins, immune complexes, and bacterial peptides.

Peroxide is the ammunition of your killer cells. Your
body's elite corps of bacterial assassins, called polymor-
phonuclear leukocytes (PMN's), engulf bacteria then kill
them with the "respiratory burst." The cell combines oxygen and water, making H_2O_2. That's the respiratory burst.
The H_2O_2 then zaps the bacteria.

Those PMN's are really smart. First they identify the
invader. (How do they do that, with no eyes and no
brain?) Then they move to the attack. (No legs, either.)
On contact, they gobble the bacteria and zap it with
H_2O_2. Amazing!

If your white cells didn't produce H_2O_2, the respiratory burst would not be possible, and bacteria would have
taken over the world a long time ago. So hydrogen peroxide has been promoted from an ordinary mouthwash to
one of life's most important bodyguards. (The Bird Man
of Alcatraz knew what he was talking about. He was a convict
who had a special love for birds. He would treat a sick bird,
who happened onto the island, with hydrogen peroxide

and had quite phenomenal results in curing his little patients. Hence his nickname, The Bird Man of Alcatraz.)

And speaking of mouthwash, don't throw that bottle of hydrogen peroxide sitting in your medicine cabinet away. It's *still* better than Scope, Lavoris, Cepacol, or any other of those red and green liqueurs peddled on TV. It kills bacteria, retards gingivitis, and reduces plaque formation. It costs about one-tenth what you'd pay for those dessert drinks. Studies have shown that Legionnaire's disease,[7] syphilis,[8] yeast (candida), viruses, and even parasites will respond to hydrogen peroxide.

Hydrogen peroxide seems to be the all-purpose executioner. The Middlesex Hospital Medical School in London experimented with H_2O_2 in the treatment of malaria, which is a parasite rather than a bacterium. They found it to be effective.[9]

Hydrogen peroxide is truly the wonder molecule. The cells in your body that fight infection, called granulocytes, produce H_2O_2 as a first line of defense against *every single type of invading organism — parasites, viruses, bacteria, and yeast. No other chemical compound comes even close to H_2O_2* in its importance to life on this earth. H_2O_2 is involved in all of life's vital processes. Protein, carbohydrate and fat metabolism, vitamin and mineral metabolism, immunity, and anything else involving life's functions require the presence of this amazing molecule.

There are over *6,100 articles* in the scientific literature dating from 1920 on the scientific applications of hydrogen peroxide. It seems inconceivable that the astounding medical cures reported in science journals over the past 75 years could have been ignored. The reasons for this scientific blindness will become apparent to you as the peroxide story unfolds.

In some mysterious way not yet identified, H_2O_2 is involved in phagocytosis, the process by which some of your blood cells eat enemy bacteria. H_2O_2 also acts like insulin, in that it aids the transport of sugar through the body.

Hydrogen peroxide may be just as important, or

more important, than thyroid for heat generation. As you know, your car won't run properly if it is cold. Neither will your body. H_2O_2, in the presence of coenzyme-Q10, creates "intracellular thermogenesis," a warming of your cells which is absolutely essential to life. As one researcher put it, the new information on H_2O_2 *affords the conceptual basis for a revolution* in our thinking about many of life's vital processes.

It's amazing how medicine has largely ignored this well-researched and unique therapy. But what's new? Some doctors still don't wash their hands between patients, although Dr. Ignatz Semilweise proved a hundred years ago that doctors were the main cause of the spread of infection in hospitals because of their contaminated hands. Nothing changes. Peroxide therapy will continue to be resisted and ridiculed by American doctors.

Most of the work at Baylor University, which we will discuss in the next chapter, was done by dripping H_2O_2 into an artery. It really isn't necessary to use the more difficult arterial route for peroxide therapy.

One of our colleagues measured a pulmonary (lung) patient's arterial pO_2 level (the measure of oxygen content), before and after hydrogen peroxide therapy. After the infusion of hydrogen peroxide, this patient's oxygen content went from 60 to 80, which is a marked improvement. You can, in fact, just look at venous blood when it's drawn from the patient following a peroxide treatment and see a marked difference in the color. It assumes the color of arterial blood, which contains more oxygen than venous blood.

Hydrogen peroxide is also necessary for the manufacture of hormone-like substances called prostaglandins. Also, hydrogen peroxide produced by ascorbic acid (vitamin C) has been shown to induce prostaglandin synthesis. This would suggest that the beneficial clinical effects observed with the use of Vitamin C in inflammatory reactions, and its protective action against infections, result from the generation of hydrogen peroxide, which in turn induces the production of prostaglandins.

Doctors at the Boston University Medical Center[10] compared the effectiveness of hyperbaric oxygen and H_2O_2 in their ability to oxygenate tissues. They put rabbits in pressure chambers and pumped in oxygen. They compared the level of tissue oxygen with the level found when H_2O_2 was given in an artery or a vein.

I'd better explain the difference between an artery and a vein — many people don't know. If you do know (or don't care), then skip the next paragraph.

The veins are the blood vessels that you see on the back of your hand, the arms and feet. You can't see arteries. The veins return the blood to the heart from the far reaches of the body. The arteries deliver the blood back to the body from the heart after it has gone through the lungs to pick up oxygen (see below).

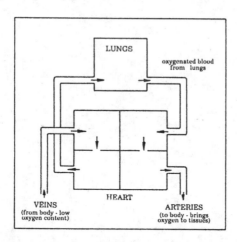

The doctors found that if they gave H_2O_2 into an artery, it was just as effective at raising tissue oxygen levels as the hyperbaric method. But given in the vein, there was no rise in oxygen levels of the tissues.

This difference is important because it is easy to give medication in a vein, but not so easy to give it through an artery. There are many reasons for this. The main one being that arteries are not as accessible as veins. It should be noted, however, that current clinical trials refute the claim that H_2O_2 doesn't work when given in the vein.

Chapter 3

The Research Proves It

In the 1960's, a team of doctors from the Baylor University Medical Center began serious study of H_2O_2 in animals, as well as humans. One of their earlier studies[1] concerned cancer therapy. Tissues are more sensitive to X-ray treatment if the oxygen supply to those tissues is maximal. Hydrogen peroxide, they reasoned, if given into a blood vessel going to the cancerous area, should make the cancer more sensitive to X-ray. Cancer cells don't like oxygen anyway, so there would be two forces working against the cancer: oxygenation and radiation. The authors reported that there appeared to be a positive effect from this combination, thus allowing effective X-ray therapy at a lower dose.

In 1964, the Baylor group did a sensational study that, again, didn't phase the medical community. Dr. Finney and his colleagues pointed out that hyperbaric oxygen therapy (getting oxygen to the tissues through increased pressure inside a chamber) was being intensely researched. But, they emphasized, the method is costly, cumbersome, and not without some danger. If oxygen could be delivered to the tissue by injecting H_2O_2 directly into blood vessels, the cost would be inconsequential compared to hyperbaric oxygen therapy. H_2O_2 therapy had long since been proven safe.

Hydrogen peroxide breaks down very rapidly on entering the bloodstream. Oxygen is released in *less than a second*. (It takes *one-tenth* of a second, to be exact.) The blood becomes supersaturated with oxygen. It's called hyperoxia. The magnitude of saturation is *far greater* than can be obtained with the expensive and cumbersome hyperbaric oxygen therapy (HBO). With HBO, two atmospheres of oxygen are about as far as they dare to go. Any pressure above that can lead to serious consequences. But with H_2O_2 therapy into a blood vessel, the oxygen delivery can be *four times* that of HBO, with no side effects whatsoever.

The Baylor researchers investigated the potential of H_2O_2 to remove the plaque of hardened arteries. Wouldn't it be sensational if they could prove that H_2O_2 would clear up the arteries like chelation therapy, but do it quicker? Chelation therapy, the dripping of agents into the veins to unplug the blood vessels, works slowly and mostly on the tiny vessels. It is an excellent therapy and will obviate the need for bypass surgery in most cases. But chelation therapy doesn't seem to affect the large vessels very much, like the big heart arteries and the aorta. It works by opening the tiny vessels at the end of the line. Wouldn't it be better if a therapy treated *all* the vessels-from the biggest to the smallest?

Finney and his colleagues have gone a long way toward proving that H_2O_2, dripped into the leg arteries of patients known to have severe arteriosclerosis, will clear those arteries of disease. When these patients died, autopsies were done to compare arteries that had been treated with H_2O_2 with those not treated. They reported: "The elution of lipids from the arterial wall by dilute hydrogen peroxide has been accomplished...." In simple English that means *the plaque buildup was removed by injecting H_2O_2* into the blood vessels. Sensational! (No one paid any attention. That was over 20 years ago.)

The investigators also reported that the improvement was not temporary. Autopsies done a year after the H_2O_2 treatments showed as much cleaning out of the arteries as in those patients who died just weeks following the procedure. Would you be willing to go in for treatment once a year or so for a simple procedure that is safe, painless, inexpensive, and effective rather than face by-pass surgery that is painful, dangerous, expensive, and at best temporarily effective? (Let me guess.)

I guess if I were a cardiac surgeon I wouldn't be very excited about this mode of therapy either. It would be like telling Chevron and Exxon we've invented a car that will run on saltwater.

In 1966, the same Baylor University group did some more interesting research with H_2O_2 and cardiac resuscitation. In fact, it was downright mind-boggling:

Victims of heart attacks often die within hours of the onset of the infarction. This is due to ventricular fibrillation, a deadly event in which the heart muscle goes crazy and beats rapidly and chaotically. This is the heart's response to oxygen-lack called hypoxia. If this dangerous "runaway heart" condition can be controlled, then the patient has an excellent opportunity to survive.

Some emergency measures have proven to be partially successful in calming the heart down, and defibrillation, an electrical shocking of the heart, has often been lifesaving. Also lidocaine, a cardiac drug given in the vein, is dramatically effective in some patients.

But remember, *the heart is responding to hypoxia,* lack of oxygen, so these methods are only of temporary benefit in most cases. If the blood could be supersaturated with oxygen, the problem would be met directly, and the patient should survive.

Hydrogen peroxide has been found to have an energizing effect on the heart muscle, causing it to beat with more vigor and efficiency (called the inotropic effect).[3] The heart exhibiting "pump failure," the inability to pump blood efficiently through the circulation, is often helped dramatically with peroxide therapy.[4] This "high output heart failure" leads to death due to backing up of fluid in the lungs, with consequent drowning. The heart is often slowed from an unhealthy, rapid rate with H_2O_2 and the blood pressure will often be appreciably reduced. "Myocardial asemia," lack of oxygen to the heart muscle, is often dramatically improved with peroxide. "Ventricular fibrillation," a totally chaotic rhythm of the heart which rapidly leads to death, has been reported to have been completely relieved with the emergency use of hydrogen peroxide.[5]

Doctor George Hart, an expert on hyperbaric oxygen at the Memorial Medical Center, Long Beach, California, tells the story of how "an elephant suddenly landed on my chest" while he was driving to the hospital one morning. He knew without a doubt that he was having a heart attack.

Doctor Hart knows what hyperbaric oxygen can do. Upon arriving at the hospital, he immediately had himself checked into a hyperbaric oxygen chamber. His chest pain was immediately relieved, and he went on to recover from his heart attack.

Unfortunately, most of us don't have access to one of these chambers. Even if they were readily available, the method would not be practical. The doctor loses access to the patient during a critical period. The treatments are expensive and the patient cannot take more than an hour to an hour and a half of treatment without getting toxic symptoms which would further complicate his condition. But oxygen delivered directly into the circulation would be another matter. This would get to the heart of the problem, pardon the expression, and immediately reoxygenate the starving heart muscle.

In their first experiment, the Baylor doctors cross-clamped the trachea of some New Zealand rabbits. In other words, they strangled them. If you can't breathe, you can't get oxygen into your blood and, thus, to the heart muscle. Within 12 minutes the rabbit will develop cardiac arrest or ventricular fibrillation and die.

Then they took another group of New Zealand rabbits (these devils are *big*— they weigh seven pounds) and gave them the same treatment. But this group was given H_2O_2 directly into the arteries of the heart. The animals were observed for *two hours* without cardiac arrest developing.

Incredible, unbelievable. Someone must repeat this experiment. If the results are the same (and I am confident they will be), then this technique, or a modification of it, should be instituted all over the nation for heart attacks.

That won't be easy. There will be three very powerful forces fighting the general acceptance of this simple therapy. First, the drug industry. H_2O_2 is not patentable. The drug industry would lose billions in lost drug sales.

Second, the FDA works in collusion with the drug industry. They can be counted on to pull every dirty trick imaginable to stop this therapy, including declaring H_2O_2 an "investigational new drug." But right now, they seem to be going in both directions.

The third force is organized medicine. In the face of these momentous experimental results, you would think that doctors would be clamoring for more information and a quick resolution as to whether the Baylor doctors know what they are talking about. You might think that would happen, but it doesn't work that way. With most doctors, it's not greed, but pride, ignorance, and bigotry that account for their resistance to new and unusual treatments.

How would *you* like it if you were a doctor and a little old lady in Adidas running shoes asked you, "Hey, Doc, what about hydrogen peroxide in the treatment of myocardial infarction, cerebro-vascular accidents, and *Clostridium Welchi* septicemia?" (You'd probably punch her out.)

Back to the experiment. Remember that first batch of giant rabbits? The ones strangled and not getting the H_2O_2? Remember that within 12 minutes they died of heart stoppage, or ventricular fibrillation? The investigators discovered, even though the animals were "in extremis" (meaning about to croak and go to that great rabbit hutch in the sky), if they were given H_2O_2, most of them would survive! Amazing — snatched back from death's door by peroxide.

Next, the researchers simulated heart attacks in the rabbits by tying off their heart blood vessels, the arteries leading to the heart muscle called coronary arteries. Ordinarily, this will lead to ventricular fibrillation and death within five to 10 minutes. Injecting H_2O_2 into a peripheral vein returned irregular heartbeats and blood pressure rapidly to normal. Even dripping the H_2O_2 directly *onto* the heart muscle, rather than *into* the bloodstream, would save the rabbit from cardiac death.

All these experiments were then repeated with pigs. The results were the same. The most remarkable observation with the pigs was that although they appeared *clinically dead* (no blood pressure and no heartbeat), *50 percent of them were revived when H_2O_2 was applied to the heart.*

The researchers next treated one human. (No strangulation was attempted this time. It's hard to find volunteers.) A 60-year-old woman developed "vascular collapse" of unknown cause. She had an abnormal heartbeat and practically no blood pressure. *Within one minute* of H_2O_2 infusion, her heart reverted to normal and blood pressure returned to a normal level.

The most hopeless area for treatment of blocked arteries is in the head and neck. The surgeons do a "roto-rooter" job on the large arteries of the neck when they are partially plugged. But it's a very dangerous procedure and will often cause what it is supposed to prevent: stroke. For the rest of the blood vessels in the head and neck — forget it. Surgical procedures have been proven worthless and currently used drugs are ineffective (or worse).

The Baylor doctors reported in 1967 a case of right vertebral artery blockage. The vertebral arteries are small, extremely important, and *totally inaccessible* blood vessels that travel from the heart, up the back of the spinal column, to the back of the brain. If one or both of these arteries become blocked you are in deep trouble. You lose speech, vision, and balance. Some victims of this type of blockage have "drop attacks." They drop to the floor just as if someone had cut their legs from under them. This happens without the slightest loss of consciousness. An inexperienced doctor will think the patient is faking because of the lack of mental change with the episode. It is a peculiar and mysterious medical phenomenon.

The Baylor case was a tough one. The patient, a 57-year-old woman who had suffered a stroke due to blockage of a large main artery in the neck, now had a blockage of the right vertebral artery.

Surgeons had operated on the blocked main vessel at the front of the neck on the right side (the right, carotid artery), with what appeared at the time to be a very successful result. But, nine months later, X-rays showed that the vertebral artery on the right was also blocked. Did the previous surgery cause this important artery in the back of the neck to plug up in a mere nine months? It is a reasonable assumption.

The patient was getting worse on drug therapy (blood thinners and cortisone), so it was elected to start her on H_2O_2 infused into the large arteries of the neck, the carotids. It was hoped that the oxygen released by the H_2O_2 would reach those tiny lifelines encased deep in bone and muscle — the vertebrals.

She had a total of 100 infusions over a period of 28 days. Within a week her coordination and speech improved, and she could sit up without dizziness.

Another thing happened with this patient that the Baylor doctors had reported previously:[6] Her blood cell count improved. Why putting H_2O_2 into the brain causes an increase in the blood elements is unknown. (One wonders what this type of treatment would do for leukemia and other blood diseases.) Subsequent to the H_2O_2 therapy, X-rays showed the vertebral artery was open, whereas before it had been tightly closed.

Remember that this was a "worst case" situation. There is not the slightest chance that anyone in vascular research would expect such a result from the simple infusion of hydrogen peroxide into the blood vessels of the neck. The outcome was simply beyond the imagination of the modern medical mind.

Animal experimentation also proved that H_2O_2 is effective rectally. Don't try this without a doctor's supervision. We don't want you to explode in the bathroom and give H_2O_2 a bad name.

Even nebulization works. Doctor Finney and his colleagues at Baylor had rabbits breathe H_2O_2 mixed in saline solution. The amount of oxygen increase found in the blood was *twice* what would be obtained from the average hyperbaric oxygen treatment. The HBO treatment costs about $150.00, the H_2O_2 nebulization, about $.10. You can see why that might upset a lot of people in the medicine business.

The chemistry is so simple that even I can understand it. Hydrogen peroxide breaks down into oxygen and water:

$$\text{catalase or}$$
$$H_2O_2 \rightarrow O_2 \text{ and } H_2O$$
$$\text{peroxidase}$$

Hydrogen Peroxide and Cancer

Radiation therapy of cancer is a two-edged sword. In many cases, the X-ray will shrink the tumor mass; but it also shrinks the patient's immune system. In other words, the treatment is successful, in that the cancerous tumor gets smaller, but you shorten the life of the patient.

There is a direct relationship between the amount of oxygen in a cancer mass (tumor) and the effectiveness of X-ray. The more oxygen present, the more lethal the X-ray to cancer cells. The hyperbaric oxygen chambers mentioned previously would probably work, but there is no way to get the X-ray to the patient if he is sealed in a tank, under pressure. A large room which also puts the X-ray equipment under pressure would have to be built. This would be prohibitively expensive, and the danger of explosion would always be present.

The Baylor team reasoned that if they put oxygen into the tumor mass by injecting H_2O_2 into the artery leading to the tumor, the tumor would be much more receptive to X-ray destruction. They studied a total of 190 patients using hydrogen peroxide infused into the artery leading to the tumorous cancer. The experiment took six years. Their results were astounding.

An 88-year-old man with a squamous cell carcinoma (a lethal cancer that is usually caused by chewing tobacco or cigarette smoking) on his right cheek mucous membrane was treated by dripping H_2O_2 into the neck artery leading to this terrible cancer. The patient was alive and *free of evidence of cancer six years later.* The life expectancy of this elderly gentleman would be, under conventional treatment, about 12 to 18 months. (Less, if he was given chemotherapy.)

A 29-year-old man had a "fungating mass under the jaw with fixation of the tongue" and gangrene of the jaw bone. In other words, a horrible, disgusting mess which would ordinarily lead to a quick demise (and the sooner the better). He was treated by the same method of H_2O_2 infusion into the cancer, combined with X-ray. At the time of the report (1967), the doctors said the patient was *alive and free of cancer.*

The researchers modestly reported: "These preliminary results suggest an improvement in the radio-therapeutic ratio."

One doctor listening to the report was flabbergasted. "You mean the tumor went down that fast? It was such a dramatic difference in size. I couldn't imagine that happening."

Chapter 4

Criticisms of Hydrogen Peroxide Therapy

Some Possible Side-Effects

Surgeons have to be a little careful in using hydrogen peroxide to irrigate deep wounds. If the H_2O_2 becomes trapped, it may go into the circulation, causing gas embolism — an oxygen bubble that can block the circulation in the lungs.

A case was reported in the *British Medical Journal* of a man with deep abscess of the thigh.[1] Three percent H_2O_2 was pumped into the wound. Then the surgeon pressed the thigh to expel the H_2O_2. Trouble is, the H_2O_2 went both ways-out of the wound opening and also into the bloodstream. The patient became blue and went into shock. He was given cortisone and blood for treatment (both ill-advised, in my opinion). But in spite of this catastrophic event and the ensuing bad treatment, the patient made a complete recovery.

This case emphasizes the safety of H_2O_2. An air embolus, which is mostly nitrogen, can be fatal or cause permanent paralysis. But a pure oxygen embolus quickly dissolves into the tissues and so rarely causes any permanent damage.

Hydrogen peroxide colitis is another potential hazard in the misuse of H_2O_2. Chemical ulcerative colitis, a serious ulceration of the large bowel causing cramping and bloody diarrhea, can be caused by H_2O_2.

Yale Medical School investigators reported three

cases of ulcerative colitis, in patients with no history of this disease, following the use of H_2O_2 in an enema.[2] All three recovered, but they were seriously ill. As the authors observed, "sepsis invariably occurs in association with hydrogen peroxide colitis." Sepsis means bacteria in the blood, a potentially fatal complication.

But, as often happens in medical reporting, the investigators opined beyond their state of knowledge, and thereby added to the store of false reporting on H_2O_2. They said in their discussion of the cases that "solutions of hydrogen peroxide are relatively weak germicides." They also remarked on the "exotic use" of H_2O_2 in the vein for treatment of blocked arteries. They claimed that the procedure was discontinued: "Potentially lethal gas embolism led to the discontinuation of such therapy." Finney and the other Baylor investigators never reported any such problems. This kind of disinformation can set a good therapy back 50 years.

The Yale doctors did conclude that peroxide enemas are safe if the concentration is carefully controlled. But that got lost in the adverse report. Govoni reported 30 cases using 10 cc of three percent H_2O_2 in one liter of water with no complications.[3]

As with any treatment, there are possible side effects with peroxide, but, fortunately, they are usually minor.

The most frequent side effect reported is inflammation of the vein through which the infusion was given. This phenomenon is very inconsistent, occurring repeatedly in some patients, but rarely in others. This reaction is less likely to occur if a large vein, such as the one in the forearm, is used for infusion and the rate of administration is slow. At least one and a half hours should be used for every treatment. For some reason not understood, inflammation of the vein may not appear until the day after the treatment. If it does occur, heat may make the reaction even more severe, since heat speeds up the rate of most biochemical reactions, and, therefore, heat is not recommended. An ice pack would be more appropriate for discomfort, but it will clear without any treatment at all.

Occasionally, a non-tender red streak will appear where the infusion is given, and a white, blanched appearance may occur in the center of the red streak. Treatments are not discontinued because of this, and there have been no adverse effects from it. This streaking, whether red or white, is not related to the inflammation of the vein mentioned previously, and there seems to be no correlation.

The treatment can be *too effective* and cause a so-called *Herxheimer* reaction. This consists of migratory aches, nausea, sometimes headaches, chills without any fever and mild diarrhea. This is due to an "overkill." The breakdown of products of the infective agent causes the reaction. It will usually occur within the first three treatments if it is going to occur at all, and, after it clears, the patient continues to improve. The *Herxheimer* reaction is not consistent and is not predictable.

There have been attempts by some entrepreneurs interested in competitive modes of therapy to frighten people away from intravenous peroxide by pointing out certain toxic reactions which, in reality, occur only in the laboratory and not in humans. These promoters will report on the dark consequences of lipid peroxidation, platelet aggregation, chromosomal aberrations, etc. Clinically, however, no significant acute toxicity has been observed in several hundred patients, some receiving up to 40 and 50 infusions of hydrogen peroxide. The treatment is quite safe when given by a qualified physician. The worst side-effect is: "Patient has deteriorated considerably since last treatment" — because he felt so well that he abruptly quit the therapy. We relate such a case on page 124.

Can You Take Hydrogen Peroxide Orally?

Dr. Edward C. Rosenow, an eminent scientist, was the first to suggest taking H_2O_2 by mouth. The formula he devised is still the standard for peroxide taken orally.

Many people are now recommending hydrogen

peroxide by mouth. It appears efficacious by mouth, but extreme caution has been advised. Ascorbate, iron, and fats in the stomach change H_2O_2 into superoxide free radicals.[4] These free radicals can do severe damage to the lining of your stomach. Studies on mice given H_2O_2, even in low concentrations, were indicative of the risk from taking H_2O_2 by mouth. The mice developed erosion of the stomach lining, tumors, and in some, cancer.

But these studies have been challenged by none other than the Food and Drug Administration (FDA).

I don't like the FDA any more than you do. Anyone who has studied the history of the FDA knows they have a very cozy relationship with the drug industry. They are now brazenly (and illegally) joined with the drug industry, the Post Office police, the AMA *(sub rosa)* and the Federal Trade Commission (FTC) in an all-out attempt to destroy the natural health movement in the U.S.

But that's what makes their defense of H_2O_2 so interesting. H_2O_2 is dirt cheap. The drug companies can't patent it, so it's a threat to the antibiotic industry (it has remarkable antibiotic effects). It's a threat to the heart bypass industry (it will clean arteries of atherosclerotic buildup), and it's a threat to the surgical and chemotherapy cancer treatment industry (combined with radiation, it will rapidly reduce cancer growths with less toxic doses of X-ray). If the FDA runs true to form, it will eventually join its brothers in the drug industry — medicine, the Post Office, and the FTC — and condemn peroxide therapy.

I have good friends who use oral H_2O_2 in their practice. I have good friends who claim that it's dangerous to use it orally. All I can do is present both sides and let you make up your own mind as to whether it's safe.

Just because it causes cancer of the stomach in mice doesn't mean it does in humans. The dose used may have been unrealistically high, as in the studies that resulted in the banning of cyclamate. Or the frequency of dosage may have been excessive. After all, it's dose times frequency that tells you how much your mouse is actually getting.

Incidentally, garlic extract, called Kyolic, will detoxify even large doses of cyclamate. It may do the same for H_2O_2; I don't know. Don't get me wrong. I'm not recommending cyclamate for your coffee. I just want to make the point that animal experimentation can be misleading.

The practitioners using H2O2 by mouth say they "haven't had any trouble." That may be like the man who jumped from the 40th floor. As he passed the 10th floor he yelled to a man looking out the window: "So far, so good!"

I'm not saying that everything is going to go splat with people taking H_2O_2 by mouth. But the evidence I have seen can't be ignored. Those mice I mentioned were given very small doses and they developed serious gastric problems, including cancer, *in as little as three weeks*. But mice aren't people.

Hydrogen peroxide reacts with fatty acids in the stomach to form hydroxyl radicals. Hydroxyl free radicals are probably one of the major factors in many degenerative diseases, including cancer. Much of the body contains enzymes that quickly break up H_2O_2 into oxygen and water. But the stomach and intestinal tract contain very little of these protective enzymes, so ulceration of the lining could theoretically develop. Ulceration can lead to hyperplasia, and hyperplasia to cancer.

From the *Federal Register,* January 9, 1981: "In response to the study from Japan, the FDA initiated a review of all available safety data on hydrogen peroxide including the Japanese study and subsequent clarification obtained from the Japanese authors. FDA concludes after this review that there is insufficient evidence from the Japanese study and elsewhere to conclude that hydrogen peroxide is a duodenal carcinogen."

My conclusion: I don't think H_2O_2 is dangerous taken orally as long as the recommended dose is not exceeded (ten drops of three percent H_2O_2, three times a day).

But *a caveat:* Dr. Charles Farr, who probably knows the research literature better than anyone, does not agree. *Recent research confirms Dr. Farr's doubts.*[5] Dr. Farr says that further evidence exists that H_2O_2 should *not* be taken by mouth, especially when there is food in the stomach. If you do take H_2O_2 orally (and this is *not* a recommendation that you do so), take it on an empty stomach.

The reagent grade H_2O_2 is probably the safest. One reason is because of the lead found in the other grades. USP peroxide, for instance, contains *five times* more lead than reagent grade. But after proper dilution, the contamination problem is revealed to be far worse. There is *200 times* more lead or other heavy metals in the other mixtures than in the reagent grade.[6] Food grade has not been tested for lead at this time, but it may very well have an even higher level; or it may not.

Occasionally, a patient will have a reaction to peroxide. This may be due to toxins being expelled by the breakup of bacteria as the H_2O_2 zaps them, causing a *Herxheimer* type of reaction, as mentioned on page 35. It will pass after a few treatments.

Skin eruptions are a particularly good sign, although distressing to the patient. This means that toxins are being released. There may even be boils or other inflammatory conditions that develop temporarily. Severe fatigue is not unusual, and there may be sleepiness, nausea, or diarrhea. The reaction will vary with the condition being treated.

None of these reactions are common, but almost any kind of minor reaction is possible. The dosage or frequency of treatment can be reduced, but *don't stop*. Eventually, you will probably be rewarded with better health. Before starting, consult a doctor familiar with the procedure. (That won't be easy. Even doctors who use it I.V. often are chary of recommending it by mouth.)

Negative Reports on H_2O_2

Not all reports have been favorable. Researchers at Duke University School of Medicine tried intravenous H_2O_2 infusions in pigs. All of the animals developed a serious blood condition called methemoglobinemia. But none of the human experiments have caused this complication.

(Just another example of how unreliable animal data can be. People aren't pigs, even though some may act like it).

Mary Beth Dodson — A Negative Report

"I had the greatest faith in it when I started," Mary Beth told me.

Mary Beth has multiple sclerosis. She had worked up to 50 drops of H_2O_2 by mouth daily, with no good effect after three months. It was causing nausea, so she gave it up.

She is the only case of multiple sclerosis I have interviewed who has not responded, at least partially, to H_2O_2. However, I would not classify her as a failure until she has tried intravenous H_2O_2. I assured her that the intravenous method would not cause nausea, and I urged her to find a doctor who uses this therapy. For a remarkable case of multiple sclerosis, see page 98.

Chapter 5

The Farr Experiments

Charles H. Farr, M.D., Ph.D., has done a benchmark experiment proving that, contrary to established opinion, oxygen given in the vein isn't dissipated in the lungs. The inset on page 21 shows a simplified version of the circulatory system. (It helped me get through medical school.) It was said that the oxygen released by H_2O_2 when given in the vein would somehow be lost, presumably in the expired air. Certainly some of it may be lost this way, but there was no logical reason to think that it would *all* be lost. And that's what Dr. Farr set out to disprove.

Patients were given H_2O_2 in an arm vein. Using high tech instruments, Dr. Farr proved: (1) The metabolic rate was significantly increased; (2) dilation of the small arteries of the body occurred; and (3) oxygen from H_2O_2 infusions did, indeed, remain in circulation and was not lost in expired air.

The test subjects reported increased mental alertness, increased visual acuity, increased brightness of surroundings, and a feeling of relaxation. Farr and his associates reported significant improvement in many acute conditions, including infection, allergy, and influenza.

The Farr group is now experimenting with combining H_2O_2 treatment with EDTA chelation therapy. The two agents cannot be mixed, because serious reaction can occur if H_2O_2 is mixed with other active compounds. Doctor Farr is inviting other qualified chelation therapists to participate in a nationwide study of this combination, called Chelox therapy. Both lay persons and physicians from across the United States and several foreign countries have formed a nonprofit organization to promote

and support further research in this new field of bio-oxidation. The organization is called the *International Oxidative Medicine Association (IOMA)*. *For more information on this
wonderful organization, please see Appendix I.*

Hydrogen Peroxide
and the Immune System

Dr. Charles Farr made an astute clinical observation that
after patients received a series of treatments with intravenous hydrogen peroxide, a sensitivity to pollen and food
allergies clinically improved. He also noted improvement
in allergic bronchitis, asthma, and chronic sinusitis. Those
observations led him to investigate the effects of intravenous hydrogen peroxide on serum antibody titres and immune globulin fractions. Other investigators have
reported that both T- and B-cells are stressed when exposed to hydrogen peroxide and that the surviving T-cells
become resistant to secondary oxidative stress, while the
B-cells remain fragile.[1]

In confirmation of this, Farr had previously reported
studies of patients receiving intravenous hydrogen peroxide who had an average of 55 percent reduction of their
null cells. Null cells are precursors, or *baby cells,* that
branch out in maturity to various cell types such as B-cells
and T-cells. The reduction in null cells is probably due to
an increase in their differentiation into T-cells and B-cells,
which are found to be increased by 20 to 35 percent
within 24 hours following the intravenous hydrogen peroxide infusion. Although the original (preinfused) population of T-cells and B-cells is reduced following the
oxidative stress of hydrogen peroxide, there is a rebound
which leads to a net increase as mentioned above.

T- and B-cells identify antigenic (foreign) substances and
produce the necessary antibodies in response to this rec-
ognition. The mechanism by which intravenous hydrogen
peroxide relieves allergy symptoms is not understood, but
it is probably due to the young, virginal T- and B-cells not
having been exposed to previous antigens, causing them

not to react against the antigens.

Patients demonstrating allergy symptoms or autoimmune diseases were randomly chosen for these studies from Farr's clinical population. Immune globulins IGG, IGA, IGM and IGE were measured before and after intravenous hydrogen peroxide treatments. The clinical improvement observed indeed corresponded to the reduction in these immune globulins.

Next, Farr studied Ebstein-Barr virus (EBV) and candida antibody titres, which were measured before and after intravenous hydrogen peroxide treatments. The patients usually received 20 weekly treatments administered as follows: one treatment a week for 10 weeks, no treatments for 30 days, and then repeat another ten-treatment series. Antibody titres were measured at the beginning, after the 20th treatment and then again at three months and six months. Clinical improvement again paralleled a reduction in antibody titres in all patients studied. The EBV patient group (chronic fatigue syndrome) had a significant improvement in energy and endurance, with a reduction in complaints of fatigue. The candida patients also were clinically improved, relative to the reduction of their candida antibody titres, by intravenous hydrogen peroxide.

In other studies of autoimmune antibodies (thought to cause Rheumatoid Arthritis, Lupus, Sclerodermia, etc.) Farr found *in all cases studied, autoimmune antibodies could no longer be detected after a series of 10 or more intravenous hydrogen peroxide treatments.* These findings support the concept that intravenous hydrogen peroxide does reduce circulation T- and B-cells, but the new population of virginal T- and B-cells derived from null cells, which have not been tagged to produce specific antibodies, modify the amount of circulating antibodies quite significantly. The modification of the circulating and immune globulins, that is, the decrease in those globulins, correlates with the clinical improvement seen in the patient.[2]

Treatment with H$_2$O$_2$ —
Some Amazing Cases from the Farr Clinic

Bronchiectasis

One of the most discouraging maladies that doctors have to treat is bronchiectasis. Bronchiectasis is basically pus pockets within the lung. These patients constantly cough foul-smelling phlegm, are short of breath, often blue in the face, and are greatly debilitated and weakened by constantly having to fight for breath. Farr reported the case of a 67-year-old woman who had suffered from the typical picture of cough and shortness of breath for about 15 years. After 20 treatments with peroxide, the patient's cough substantially subsided, and she was no longer producing bloody sputum. She was also breathing with much less difficulty.

Hardening of the Arteries — Heart Disease

Mr. J.H. was being treated at the clinic of Dr. Charles H. Farr in Oklahoma City for heart disease. He had received 11 treatments of chelation.

On the way to the clinic for his 12th treatment, he developed signs of a stroke. His speech became slurred, his vision blurred and there was drooling from the side of the mouth. When Dr. Farr examined him at the office, the patient was confused and disoriented. This 71-year-old gentleman was obviously in serious trouble.

Very few doctors would have had the courage to do what Dr. Farr did next. Rather than packing him off to the hospital and turning the responsibility of the case over to a neurologist (who would have had nothing definitive to offer the patient), Dr. Farr immediately started an intravenous infusion of H$_2$O$_2$.

Within 15 minutes, the patient's mind cleared and his speech improved. *Within one hour, his symptoms had gone away entirely.* This case was phenomenal.

The following case can only be described as miraculous:

J.O. was a 67-year-old man with severe blockage of the

arteries to his legs and extensive blockage of the vessels in his heart. He had endured bypass operations on both legs and a four-vessel bypass on his heart. This was a terminally ill man ravaged with arteriosclerosis. All of his tissues were literally starving for oxygen.

His surgeons offered little hope. He had gangrene, a rotting of tissue due to lack of oxygen, and the surgeons said an amputation of the left leg below the knee was necessary. If he refused the surgery, they would have to operate later and take off the entire leg — fix it now, or pay more later.

J.O. had been taking chelation therapy from another physician in New Jersey, who referred him to Dr. Farr. The results had been disappointing. Pain in his big toe was excruciating and constant. Willing to try anything within reason, J.O. agreed to let Dr. Farr try daily intravenous H_2O_2 therapy.

Twenty-four hours after the first treatment his pain had decreased, and by the fourth intravenous, had almost disappeared. The inflamed tissue cleared rapidly, and he put away his crutches. Eventually, he did lose a toe, but his leg was saved.

Temporal Arteritis

You may have never heard of temporal arteritis, but if you ever get it, you'll never forget the experience. It's characterized by severe pain and tenderness to touch at the main superficial artery of the temple. If it is not diagnosed promptly, it can lead to blindness.

M.G., a 71-year-old woman, developed temporal arteritis in 1960. She suffered for years before the condition was properly diagnosed. Fortunately, she did not go blind, and with cortisone treatment, she got relief.

But, as with most drugs, cortisone is a two-edged sword. She developed ulcers, an inflamed pancreas, and colitis. She had traded one terrible disease for three.

M.G. was given chelation therapy and her symptoms gradually cleared. She did well until 1985, when the dreaded headaches of temporal arteritis returned. She needed cortisone again, but that was obviously out of the question because of her severe previous reaction to it.

Dr. Farr recommended a trial of H_2O_2 therapy, because peroxide had proven of value in many inflammatory processes such as pneumonia and asthma. Temporal arteritis is an inflammation of the temporal artery, so, he reasoned, H_2O_2 should be of value.

She was started on an intravenous drip of peroxide, and, within a few hours, she was considerably relieved. After a second infusion a week later, she was completely well.

Shingles (Varicella Zoster)

I have seen patients in such severe pain from shingles that they had contemplated suicide. Shingles is an inflammation of the nerve endings caused by the chicken pox virus. Ugly and painful blisters appear on the skin along the distribution of a nerve from the spine. Many treatments have been tried for this debilitating condition, most of them unsatisfactory. The pain of shingles may go on for years, ruining an otherwise happy old age.

Dr. Farr treated a 69-year-old man with severe shingles on his neck, shoulder, and right arm. Three days after the H_2O_2 infusion, he was noticeably better, and in one week he was pain free. The ugly, bluish blisters were rapidly drying up.

Dr. Farr remarked: "We have treated shingles with many different therapeutic modalities with varying success. Using H_2O_2 as a therapeutic tool in this case brought about resolution two to three times faster than any modality we have previously employed."

It doesn't always work.

Chronic Obstructive Pulmonary Disease (COPD)

COPD is not curable. Ask any lung specialist. The treatment is largely a garbage collector's operation and a continual fight to keep the bronchial tubes open. The *garbage*

I refer to is the mucous and pus that constantly threatens to block the respiratory passages and kill the patient. Scarring, as a result of the chronic inflammation and spasm of the bronchial passages, adds to the problem.

There may be hope for these miserable people — if the following case turns out to be the norm.

C.G. had a long history of COPD. When seen at the Farr Clinic she was rapidly deteriorating. She was constantly coughing up yellow phlegm and had bluish lips — a sign of serious oxygen deprivation. These are the cases you hate to see come in the office. It's enough to give even a doctor humility.

She was started on intravenous H_2O_2, which, in a few minutes, precipitated severe coughing and the expelling of yellow mucous. This coughing and mucous production could be turned off and on by simply turning the H_2O_2 drip off and on.

Dr. Farr terms this *effervescent debridement*. The oxygen seeps into the air pockets under the mucous layer and literally bubbles the mucous up the respiratory passages. The rising mucous irritates the bronchial passage, causing a cough which acts as a *booster rocket*, and so, out comes the junk. That's Farr's theory. It makes sense to me.

This patient received additional dividends from the therapy. She had suffered from chronic diarrhea for over two years. This promptly cleared, as did her migratory arthritis and muscle pain.

The Yeast Syndrome

It seems that everybody who goes to the doctor's office these days thinks he has *candida*. A large percentage of them are right. Most respond to nystatin and candida extract injections. But some are very difficult to treat. Nothing works.

P.M. had received repeated treatments for chronic polysystemic candidiasis over a period of five years. Her story and her symptoms are classic for the yeast syndrome.

The symptoms started after prolonged treatment

with antibiotics for lung infections. She had chronic vaginal yeast infection, intermittent diarrhea, fatigue, acne (although she was 34 years old), arthritis, headaches, and difficulty concentrating.

She had been tried on all of the known therapies for yeast: diet, nystatin, acidophilus, caprylic acid, homeopathics, herbs, yeast extract injections for desensitization, and ketoconazole (Nizoral). She would improve temporarily on each treatment and then the symptoms would return.

P.M. became incapacitated and totally dependent on her mother. She became so debilitated that she could hardly dress herself.

After two intravenous H_2O_2 treatments administered by Dr. Farr, she reported a significant improvement in alertness and ability to concentrate, and she had an increased feeling of well-being. Her acne improved rapidly, as did her strength. *After eight treatments, she was free of symptoms for the first time in eight years.* When seen two months later, she showed no signs of candidiasis, and her allergy to yeast was markedly diminished by skin test. For the tough yeast problem, it looks like H_2O_2 therapy is the answer.

Flu Syndrome

Probably the condition for which H_2O_2 will find its greatest use is with flu and other acute respiratory infections.

A 67-year-old man came to the Farr Clinic complaining of fever, chills, sore throat, cough and aching in the bones for 12 hours; a typical case of viremia, the flu, or, in popular parlance, the crud.

He was placed on an H_2O_2 drip. His temperature was 102 at the beginning of the treatment. The next day his temperature was down to 101, and another treatment was given. *Before the infusion was finished,* his temperature had returned to normal and he was completely free of symptoms. The following day he returned to work and remained well.

One of my patients, a beautiful model, was scheduled to go to Dallas in two days for an assignment. She came in with red eyes, a runny red nose, and a fever of 101. Things did not seem promising for her trip. Models are no longer models when they have red noses and red eyes.

She was started on a peroxide drip and given 10 mg of Coenzyme Q10 by mouth to help the oxygen delivery. The next morning she was 90 percent well, and the following morning, the day for departure to Dallas, she was completely well.

We could relate many similar "flu stories," but it would be monotonous reading: first day sick, second day 90 percent well, and third day back to normal. I have never seen anything like it.

Can you imagine the millions of lost man-hours (woman-hours, too) that will be saved if this treatment becomes popular? (Nyquil and Bayer Aspirin Co. aren't going to like it.)

Most of the previous work done with H_2O_2 used the arterial route, the blood vessels carrying oxygenated blood *to the tissues*. (If confused, go back to the diagram on page 21.) It was postulated that giving H_2O_2 in the vein, i.e., the blood vessels returning blood to *the heart and lungs*, would cause all of the oxygen released by the H_2O_2 to be expelled by the lungs. Some previous studies appeared to confirm this hypothesis.

Fortunately for the sick and dying of this world, Dr. Charles H. Farr questioned this hypothesis, even in the face of the experiments that appeared to confirm it. How could he be getting such good results, if all the oxygen was being expelled by the lungs, he reasoned.

It had been noted in many previous experiments that H_2O_2 given in an artery, and thus delivered directly to the tissues, did not cause a rise in tissue oxygen levels until *40 minutes after the infusion*. This indicates, Dr. Farr said, that the H_2O_2 infused into the veins does not immediately break down into H_2O and O_2, and, thus, the O_2 would *not* be immediately blown out of the lungs. This means that the H₂O₂ would be distributed all over the body before releasing the O₂, and *little, if any*, would be lost through the expired air.

Dr. Farr did some simple but very convincing experiments to prove his hypothesis. If you plan to take H₂O₂ therapy, then you should understand some of the principles involved. You will see, if you understand the basics, the importance of taking your temperature during the treatments.

In the first experiment, Dr. Farr uses an oxygen-measuring instrument to measure the oxygen consumption. The subject wears a mask over his face and a delicate, computerized instrument does the rest. The machine calculates the inspired oxygen and the expired oxygen and reports the difference. The weight of the patient being known, the rate that the body is burning fuel (oxygen) can be easily determined. It's sort of like miles per gallon with your car, except we call it metabolic rate.

If the metabolic rate goes up with H₂O₂ therapy, then Farr is right, and more oxygen is getting to the tissues — *oxygenation of tissues is the name of the game for good health and longevity.*

The results of this experiment were unequivocal. In less than two minutes after the beginning of the infusion the metabolic rate began to rise. The rate of metabolism went up *100 percent* and stayed at that level until the infusion was stopped. The rate returned to pre-treatment levels in about 30 minutes.

The other experiment involved the measuring of the change in body surface temperature as a result of expansion of the tiny blood vessels in the skin (vasodilation). If the temperature goes up during the H₂O₂ infusion, then the body's oxygenation has increased and vasodilation has occurred. If the blood vessels dilate, the circulation improves and, again, more vital oxygen is getting to the tissues. Within five to 10 minutes after starting the infusion, the body surface temperature goes up by one degree, corresponding to the increase in oxygen consumption and vasodilation.

A sensitive little photo-electric cell was placed at the end of the index finger to measure the pulse *volume*. This is an accurate assessment of the expansion of the tiny blood vessels throughout your body. There was a clear and sustained increase of the pulse volume throughout the treatment.

All of these measurements — the oxygen consumption, the temperature rise, and the blood vessel dilation — were duplicated for six consecutive days on all patients. That doesn't leave much room for coincidence. In fact, the essence of scientific proof is that your results can be consistently repeated in a high percentage of cases studied. *One hundred percent repeatability* is not too bad.

So now you can see the importance of these experiments in your own case. By simply taking your temperature in the armpit and pulse volume at the finger tip we can tell if (1) the H_2O_2 we are using still has it's potency (the solution can deteriorate), and (2) is the H_2O_2 having the desired effect of oxygenation of tissue in your body.

There are very few treatments in medicine where the results can be so readily and easily determined as with peroxide. This gives peroxide therapy a tremendous advantage over any other form of treatment. Either it's working or it isn't. There is usually no in-between.

Dr. Farr made another brilliant observation from his studies. He perceived that the tiny amount of oxygen actually delivered to the tissues couldn't possibly explain the doubling of the metabolic rate observed. He calculated that it would take approximately *416 quarts* of oxygen to cause the increase in oxygenation (metabolic rate) observed in the patients. Even if the infusion was continued for 24 hours, only *three and a half quarts* of oxygen would be *produced — less than one percent* of the amount necessary to obtain the results measured.

He concluded, therefore, that the increase in oxygenation is due to the infused H_2O_2 stimulating the body's enzyme systems. So the objections being heard from scientists that only a trivial amount of oxygen could be getting to the tissues is incorrect. They are *technically* correct, but the results speak for themselves and vindicate Dr. Farr's landmark research.

The Farr research also disputes earlier findings about chemical changes in the blood. It had been reported that intravenous administration of peroxide did not change the blood elements or the chemistry of the blood. However, Farr found a significant decrease in cholesterol, triglycerides, red and white cells, potassium, sodium, calcium, iron, and most everything else.

In 12 hours, all elements had returned to a level *above* the pretreatment level, particularly the white cells. This Immune Rebound Phenomenon, a phrase coined by Dr. Farr, indicates a strong stimulation of the immune (defense) system. This helps explain why the H2O2 treatments are effective in all types of infectious diseases, i.e., influenza, allergies, candida, Ebstein-Barr, CMV, herpes, etc. Dr. Farr and his group are currently studying the effects of H2O2 in AIDS, hepatitis, encephalitis, and other serious viral diseases. Repeated infusions, as often as every day for as long as three weeks, have produced no serious

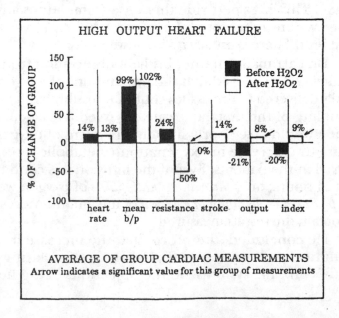

HIGH OUTPUT HEART FAILURE

AVERAGE OF GROUP CARDIAC MEASUREMENTS
Arrow indicates a significant value for this group of measurements

side effects, such as blood pressure, pulse, or respiration changes. No serious side effects have been observed in hundreds of cases treated when the H_2O_2 was properly administered.

Chapter 6

Throw Out Your Toothpaste

In the never ending fight to save our teeth, there is
nothing more useless than toothpaste. If you've been
a subscriber for any length of time, you already know
the dangers associated with fluoride use. And you also
know that it's difficult to find a toothpaste that doesn't
contain fluoride.

Yet, dentists warn that young children should not use
fluoridated toothpaste "without supervision." That is because toothpaste is sweet and children swallow it. When
they swallow it, they get *massive overdoses* of fluoride, which
is an enzymatic poison.

Whereas your water has only been contaminated
from one to ten parts per million, toothpaste contains 1000
parts per million. There is also evidence that toothpaste
can cause ulcerative colitis.

If there is one thing the American people believe in,
it's the power of toothpaste to prevent tooth decay and
gum disease. But most people don't realize that this im-
puted power of prevention defies all the known facts of
microbiology, to say nothing of common sense.

But the power of persuasion is alive and well in the
United States. Thanks to advertising, American dentists
(and their patients) are sold on the combination of the
toothbrush, toothpaste, and dental floss. In Finland it's
the toothbrush in combination with toothpicks. (Some
people have been so over sold on the virtues of tooth-
brushing that dentists now have a new industry: replacing
the enamel on teeth that has been worn away from excessive brushing.) The water pick was much in vogue in the

U.S., but in spite of being a good method for removing food particles from the spaces between the teeth and under the gums, the pick seems to have lost favor with the dentists.

None of the above is really the answer to gum and dental health, because none of these methods meet the problem of oral pathology of either the gums or the teeth. The common assumption is that particles of food rot near the teeth and thus cause a decay of the tooth surface or infection of the apposed gum, or both.

This assumption has never been proven to be true. In fact, the evidence shows just the opposite — that cavities aren't caused by rotten food. They are caused by a rotten diet. The great nutritionist, Dr. Weston Price, proved many years ago that native tribes in the South Pacific that have not been exposed to modern food do not get cavities or gum disease. His work was confirmed by Vilhjalmur Stefansson, a great Arctic explorer back in the first half of this century whose observations of the Eskimo tribes and study of the ancient skulls in Iceland showed no signs of tooth decay.

Stefansson had some penetrating words of wisdom for the overrated profession of dental hygiene: "Teeth superior on the average to those of the presidents of our largest toothpaste companies are found in the world today, and have existed in past ages, among people who violate every precept of current dentifrice advertising.... The best teeth and the healthiest mouths were found among people who ... never in their lives tasted or tested any of the other things which we usually recommend for sound teeth.... They never took any pains to cleanse their teeth or mouths. They did not visit their dentist twice a year or even once in a lifetime...."

Stefansson wrote this colorful attack back in 1936. Since then, there has been an enormous increase in the consumption of toothpaste because of the relentless propaganda from the American Dental Association (which has a vested interest in Crest — the "ADA-approved" dentifrice) and the toothpaste industry ("brush your teeth twice a day and see your dentist twice a year"). A few years after Stefansson's attack on the toothpaste industry and the dental profession, a brilliant clinician, Dr. Emanuel Libman, suggested that toothpaste might be involved in the etiology of Crohn's disease, also known as regional ileitis (President Eisenhower had it).

Regional ileitis is an inflammation of the part of the small intestine where it connects with the large intestine (colon). The area becomes scarred and an intestinal obstruction often develops. This may require emergency surgery to correct.

No one paid much attention to Libman (geniuses have that problem) because it was assumed that the mammalian gastrointestinal tract does not absorb particles such as the aluminum and silicon found in toothpaste. But doctors at the University of London have found, in experiments on rats, that polystyrene particles are indeed absorbed into the veins of the intestinal tract and reach the liver. Polystyrene is a completely insoluble substance; if it can be absorbed by the intestine, there are probably few, if any, substances that cannot enter the venous or lymphatic circulations to some degree — including aluminum and silicon.

Parenthetically, many pharmaceuticals — in fact, most of them — contain "insoluble" additives. If you are a chronic user of any medication, prescription or over-the-counter, you are a candidate for Crohn's disease. The doctors at the University of London who did the polystyrene experiments concluded: "Perhaps we should be more concerned about the fate of insoluble materials in toothpaste and pharmaceuticals which might be taken chronically." Another British group at St. Bartholomew's Hospital has added corroborating evidence by discovering aluminum, silicon, and titanium in the lesions of Crohn's disease.

It is interesting to note that regional ileitis is more common among the higher socioeconomic groups. These are the folks who are more likely to take the advice of doctors and dentists seriously and thus are more susceptible to the propaganda of the tooth fairies of the ADA.

Action to Take

1. Throw out all the toothbrushes and toothpaste in your bath room. I realize that most of you are not willing to do this, so if you must brush, get three percent hydrogen peroxide from the drug store and mix it with baking soda. Make a thick solution with it, not a paste — and brush with that. If you insist upon brushing your teeth with store-bought toothpaste, don't use any that has fluoride in it. All natural toothpaste can be purchased at most health food stores.

2. Water-pick your teeth with three percent hydrogen peroxide before bed time. See my **Final Note** below for further explanation.

3. Your toothbrush is one of the dirtiest things in your bathroom. If you use a toothbrush, dip it in three percent hydrogen peroxide after each use.

4. As I've said before, take everything in your kitchen or bath labeled as containing fluoride, pack it up, and send it to someone you hate.

5. For "mouth freshness" in the morning, rinse with three percent hydrogen peroxide. It lasts longer than Scope, Listerine, or Crest and actually kills pathogenic bacteria; the others do not. You might also try chewing on a piece of parsley.

Final Note: It is not possible for a toothbrush, a toothpick, dental floss, or a combination of all three, to remove microscopic particles of food from all of your teeth interfaces and from under your gums. That's why I never believed "oral hygiene" had much to do with preventing tooth decay.

What I'm getting at here is that if you can't rid yourself of the fear of food, and you really think your mouth has to be squeaky clean after eating, then use a water pick with three percent hydrogen peroxide after dinner. Don't worry about breakfast and lunch — the food isn't going to rot before bed time.

Another choice for the compulsive mouth cleaner is the new ultrasound toothbrush. Now *that* is industrial grade cleaning and I think it is safe — although I have seen no studies on it.

After following this regimen, your teeth will *still* rot if your diet is loaded with sugar, fluoride, heated saturated vegetable fats, and other nutrition-free food substitutes. The water pick and the ultrasound can clean your mouth but it can't clean your blood.

Hydrogen Peroxide and the Gum Doctors

They're called periodontists, but that's just a fancy name for gum doctors, the dentists who have carved a specialty out of gum diseases. You know the line they use: "Your teeth are okay, but your gums have got to go."

But a renegade doctor, Paul Keyes, says that most gum surgery is a racket and a rip-off. Doctor Keyes doesn't put it quite that bluntly, but his message is clear: "The controversy comes from people who like to do surgery and whose egos or income are threatened." His method of treating infected gums costs about $500.00. The periodontist's bill can be as high as $10,000.00. You can see why the periodontists might not like the new method.

Actually, it's not new. A reference is made to the use of hydrogen peroxide in dentistry in 1746. It was recommended for the treatment of pus pockets around the teeth, to be followed by excision of the dead tissues. One doctor commented: "The proposed treatment was all right in a high class practice where people could afford the fees; but it seemed unattainable to ordinary people, among whom one often found the worst cases." (Nothing has changed.)

The treatment consists of rubbing a mixture of baking soda and hydrogen peroxide into the gums. It's not quite that simple. The dentist has to do some housecleaning around your mouth, and the patient has to take the time at home for the peroxide to do the job. But the treatment is basically very simple and very effective.

Doctor Gerald Kramer, a Boston periodontist, is very critical, in fact, downright sarcastic, about the peroxide method. He says: "Keyes' technique is dramatized as the silver bullet which the public thinks it can use to cure gum disease at home in order to avoid those bad people who want to operate."

Sounds like a good idea to me. Dr. Jerry Garner, a gastroenterologist (gut doctor) from the National Institute of Health, would agree. He was told by a periodontist that all of his teeth would have to be removed. He went to Dr. Keyes *and six years later still had all of his teeth.*

Delores Dinapoli is another typical case. "Two years ago I went to a butcher who cut up one-fourth of my mouth. Another periodontist suggested still more surgery, but I couldn't face it. After treatment with (H_2O_2) my gums don't bleed or taste of pus. I have no pain or swelling."

Dr. Paul Cummings of Wilmington, North Carolina, is not just your ordinary dentist. He *taught* gum surgery at the University of North Carolina. Now he is a convert and reports a *98 percent success rate* in 1,000 patients using hydrogen peroxide.[1]

"The irony is that you can get better results without surgery," Cummings said. "I've been using the nonsurgical technique for five years and the results are 300 percent better than I ever got with surgery."

Cummings points out that not one clinical study has ever shown periodontal surgery to be necessary.

Dr. Kramer is right. You can usually avoid "those bad people who want to operate."

Bad Breath —
It's Most Likely From Your Nose

We used to think bad breath was primarily a matter of a moldy tongue, a rotten tooth, or something returning from your stomach. All of these things can be factors, but the most important source of bad breath is probably the sinuses, the nose, and the nasopharynx — that area your tongue won't reach, back of your nose and above the base of your tongue. The sinuses, those holes in your head bone below your eyes, are a very likely culprit for bad breath — there's *snot* up there that can get infected and rancid. The best treatment for this type of halitosis is H_2O_2. Take the drugstore variety, which is three percent; dilute it 50 percent with water and put five to ten drops in each nostril — sniff it up vigorously (it will burn a little). Do this twice daily and see if it helps. If it doesn't, then your problem is not your sinuses.

Chapter 7

Some Random Tidbits on H_2O_2

You would think that extra inspired oxygen, which is almost routine in hospitals with severely ill patients, would enhance hydrogen peroxide therapy and, therefore, oxygen consumption. After all, peroxide converts to oxygen, so more oxygen should be even better.

It doesn't seem to work that way, and the oxygen by nasal cannula or face mask may be doing more harm than good. It seems to interfere with the "respiratory burst" that we told you about (page 18).[1] If the peroxide can't convert to oxygen through the respiratory burst, then you will have a net loss of oxygen to the tissues. That's why patients on nasal oxygen must take off the oxygen during intravenous peroxide therapy.

People drink coffee in the morning because it makes them feel good. But it's not just caffeine that gives the boost. Roasting coffee beans gives them a hydrogen peroxide generating system.[2] Prepared in the usual manner, coffee will produce 750 micrograms of H_2O_2. The longer it sits, the more peroxide it produces for up to 24 hours! (I always said coffee wasn't so bad.)

Peroxide may be the greatest breakthrough we've ever had for brain tumors. Surgery destroys brain tissue, and chemotherapy for brain neoplasms is just plain quackery. Neuroblastoma cells, a virulent brain cancer, were inhibited by H_2O_2 in lab experiments.[3]

Researchers have found that, for some reason, the addition of copper to peroxide increases the lethality of peroxide on bacteria by *3,000-fold.*[4] It would be interesting to give a little copper with peroxide in a case of severe infection. We'll try it.

Fluorescent light has an adverse effect on human tissues exposed to peroxide.[5] I doubt that the fluorescent lights in a treatment room would be close enough to the infusion bottles being used to cause any problem.

An indication that peroxide therapy may help leukemia patients is the work of Maallen and Fletcher. They found that patients with leukemia had a 70 percent reduction in H_2O_2 production by their white blood cells.[6] Maybe cancer is a *peroxide deficiency*.

If you can't afford the time and money for the intravenous peroxide treatment for your cold, try this procedure: Put four ounces of 35 percent peroxide in a gallon of water. Run a cold humidifier in your bedroom all night with this mixture. My informant says that your cold will be gone in the morning.

I would consider it negligence at best and malpractice at worst not to use hydrogen peroxide in urinary drainage bags following surgery. Catheters in the bladder are notorious for causing infection. The bacteria multiply in the drainage bag and migrate up the tube into the bladder. This bacterial invasion can lead to many complications, including bacteremia and death.

Studies have shown that the addition of 30 milliliters of three percent H_2O_2 to the collection bag will keep the urine bacteria-free for eight hours.[7] If you are facing surgery and will need a catheter, encourage your doctor to order peroxide for the collection bag.

Schlegel proved beyond a doubt that you can oxygenate with hydrogen peroxide. He put some micro-organisms under a 100 percent nitrogen environment. This exclusion of oxygen ordinarily would lead to a quick death. But he bubbled in H_2O_2, and the organisms lived just as normally as cells in a natural environment.[8]

Contradictory reports continue to be published. An article in *Infection & Immunity* (June 1985)[9] concluded that peroxide infusions in rabbits didn't have any effect on infection. Hydrogen peroxide doesn't work at all to protect the heart of rats. In fact, it does more harm than good. (But who cares?)

It just shows you how rat experiments can be misleading. Makes you wonder how many good things may have been put aside because they didn't work in rats. On the other hand, some things that work just fine in rats turn out to be lethal to people, like the great AZT experiment on AIDS. It works great on animals but drives humans crazy — then they die.

Hydrogen peroxide has led the way, but modern science may have produced something even better. The Japanese have invented a blood substitute called Flusol that may replace H_2O_2 therapy. Flusol is being used experimentally for cancer radiation therapy in place of peroxide.

DMSO has long been an interest of mine, so I was delighted to find some research that combined DMSO with H_2O_2 in the treatment of cardiovascular disease. Baylor University was again the pioneer institution.[10]

The Baylor investigators found that DMSO, combined with peroxide, worked better in protecting the heart from blockage (heart attack) than using peroxide alone. Their statistics weren't all that convincing, but the experiment was. Eight of the nine pigs survived the heart attack with H_2O_2 treatment alone, and eight of nine also survived when DMSO was added to the peroxide. But when the heart muscle was examined under the microscope, the combined DMSO-H_2O_2 treatment group showed significantly less damage to the heart muscle.

One reason interest in H_2O_2 as a therapeutic agent waned is because animal experiments were often negative or contradictory. Dr. Lorencz, from the University of Chicago, for instance, found that intravenous peroxide therapy didn't add oxygen to the system in dogs, rats, and roosters. That's why you have to be very careful in projecting animal results to humans.

Humans, cats, and horses respond well to H_2O_2 because their blood contains catalase, the enzyme necessary to convert H_2O_2 into water and oxygen. (Your pet goat won't respond to peroxide. Neither will your pet chicken, but your pet fish will.)

Lorencz reasoned that hydrogen peroxide should be safer than intravenous oxygen because, *since the hydrogen peroxide is in solution, molecules of it are widely separated from each other by water.* The bubbles, he surmised, would be minute and very unlikely to cause a dangerous gas embolism.

First, Lorencz experimented by putting peroxide in beakers of human, cat, dog, rabbit, chicken, and rat blood. In all of the animals except the chicken and the dog, the blood with peroxide added retained the bright red color of oxygen-rich blood. As was expected, the dog and chicken blood remained dark, indicating low oxygen content. The peroxide in the dog and chicken blood had not broken down into oxygen and water because there was none of the enzyme, catalase, present to decompose the H_2O_2.

Lorencz made another important observation, which I can verify from the frightening experience of a colleague of mine. Dr. Lorencz found that there is a large variation in the susceptibility of various animal species to bubble formation (embolization) from the oxygen of hydrogen peroxide given intravenously. Lorencz also found that there is a considerable variation within the same species, including man.

My colleague, Dr. X, will attest to *that.* Dr. X was treating a very prominent person with ozone intravenously. Ozone, O_3, is another way to deliver oxygen to the tissues. But bubbling, i.e., emboli, is more likely to occur with this type of therapy. The patient went into convulsions halfway through the treatment.

Can you imagine my friend's consternation at seeing this famous woman having a fit in his office? He immediately instituted proper emergency care, and she quickly recovered without harm.

And the great news here is that *she was not really in danger,* even though she had a seizure. Lorencz found that even if animals were driven to a serious stage of collapse with peroxide, just discontinuing the therapy was all the treatment they needed. He reported *rapid and complete recovery ... even at near terminal stages,* when the treatment was discontinued. That's because the oxygen bubbles dissolve very rapidly. The *doctor* may die of a fright-induced stroke, but the patient will be okay.

Now that hydrogen peroxide is replacing ozone therapy, convulsions simply don't occur.

Ozone had its place and may still have uses in surgery. A Dr. Wolfe used it during World War I for infected shrapnel wounds by placing a silk bag over the infected tissue and pumping ozone into it. His good results were reported in the German medical journals of the '20s.

Siderova's research in 1944[11] proved that peroxide infusions work remarkably well against cyanide poisoning. So H_2O_2 eliminates another expensive and cumbersome hyperbaric oxygen therapy. But the hyperbaric oxygen chamber still has its place. Carbon monoxide (CO) poisoning, effectively treated by hyperbaric oxygen, is not treatable by peroxide. Dr. Farr says that he's not convinced peroxide won't work in CO-poisoning.

Dr. Lorencz then tried to treat various forms of chemical toxic shock with peroxide. It didn't work. Also, he reported, severe blood loss didn't respond to hydrogen peroxide therapy. But remember, this research was done on cats. Humans carry around a lot of catalase enzyme, and it might work on humans dying from hemorrhage. I think it would work, and it should be tried in emergency situations. With the present problem of blood transfusions and AIDS, *anything* reasonable should be tried.

Hydrogen Peroxide and the Food Revolution

A lot of farmers (and people who make their living from farmers) are doing a lot of hand-wringing about the farmer's plight. You wouldn't expect hydrogen peroxide to have anything to do with helping the farmer, but it's going to help the smart ones.

It has been discovered that corn cobs, straw, plant stalks, and other vegetable waste can be made into edible animal feed by treatment with hydrogen peroxide. Just imagine — a pile of useless corn stalks and weeds turned into animal feed. This will drastically reduce the cost of beef, milk, and other animal products. The straw or other waste is simply soaked in H_2O_2 for a few hours, and presto-food. The H_2O_2 makes the straw digestible and nutritionally enhanced. It's just as good or better than corn, which is expensive.

People who worry about population explosion and starvation are ecstatic about turning waste into food to feed the starving millions. They are wrong, of course. First, the population explosion is largely a media event and a myth. Second, starvation is not caused by lack of food. Starvation is caused by a lack of freedom. You rarely see people starving in a free country.

Anyway, there's a lot more to the peroxide-food story. But you get the idea. It's a momentous advance in food technology.

Before Cooking Fish, Give it a Hydrogen Peroxide Bath

The Consumers Union did a study of sanitary conditions and the state of the fish supply at markets around the U.S. What they found was far worse than a three-day-old dead fish and they raised a stink about it all the way to Washington.

From *Consumer Reports*: "Nearly half the fish we tested was contaminated by bacteria from human or animal feces ... for nearly 25 percent of our samples the bacteria count exceeded the upper limits of our test methods."

In all, half the fish was found to be rotten or "semi-rotten" and so unfit for human consumption. *Consumer Reports* added sardonically: "When bacteria counts hit ten million (colonies per gram) or more, fish should be headed for the grave rather than the dinner plate."

Perhaps rotten is too harsh an indictment here. Much of the bacteria is *surface* contamination and can be removed by wiping the surface of the fish carefully after rinsing in three percent hydrogen peroxide.[12]

The Water You Drink

Back in the 1970's, people didn't worry about their water. They trusted the water company. And, after all, motor oil is motor oil and water is water. It may taste like it came out of your swimming pool, but it wouldn't hurt you. That was contemporary logic. People trusted chemicals.

I had been warning people in Florida, where I practiced at the time, that they shouldn't drink the municipal water. Research had shown that chlorine causes cancer. The chlorine reacts chemically with organic (plant and animal) materials to form cancer-causing products called trihalomethanes.

In Douglas County, Georgia, the water has so much chlorine in it that the county warned people not to use it in their swimming pools until it was treated. *But they didn't tell them not to drink it.*

If your water comes from rivers or reservoirs (and most of it does) rather than wells, the problem is even worse. This surface water reacts with chlorine to form chloroform, a highly carcinogenic substance.

I told people about this on my nutrition radio program. The medical profession didn't take kindly to a doctor alarming people about their water. They said I was irresponsible and just trying to get some attention (I was innocent of charge one and guilty of charge two).

Less than six weeks after I dropped the cancer bombshell on my radio listeners, the front-page headline in the Miami *Herald* read: *Chlorine in water linked to cancer.*

I didn't get an apology from the medical society.

Belle Glade, Florida is a peculiar place. It's not the end of the world, but you can see it from there. They have heat, humidity, mosquitoes, roaches, flies, gnats, rattlesnakes, water moccasins, a high incidence of AIDS, and a very high level of trihalomethanes from the lousy water they take from Lake Okeechobee. Not your basic paradise.

Is it a coincidence that they have the highest per capita incidence of AIDS in the country and also the highest level of trihalomethanes in their water?

Hydrogen peroxide to the rescue. Emery Industries of Cincinnati, Ohio is installing its first major ozone treatment system in Belle Glade. Ozone is O_3. It breaks down into water and oxygen (H_2O and O_2) just like hydrogen peroxide.

The Europeans were way ahead of us on ozone. Now the European companies are moving into the U.S. market. With all our technology, you wonder how we could be so far behind Europe in water technology and water nutrition. Ozone not only kills bacteria, but it also destroys viruses and parasites. Instead of *causing* a bad smell and taste, like chlorine, it removes all odors and taste. Are Europeans smarter than us? They certainly are when it comes to water.

Ozonized water won't be therapeutic and nutritious like lithia water, but it will beat distilled water for your coffee and soup.[13]

Jump-Starting Your Thyroid Gland

The rise in body temperature during peroxide therapy undoubtedly reflects stimulation of the thyroid gland, as well as stimulation of the immune system. We monitor the effectiveness of thyroid hormone by periodically checking the body temperature. As the thyroid starts working, the temperature slowly rises. It usually takes about eight weeks to see the effect and measure a temperature rise of a few tenths of a degree.

But with the peroxide therapy, a *full degree* temperature change occurs in about *15 minutes* instead of eight weeks.

Because of this dramatic change, we now recommend to our patients starting on thyroid that they *jump-start* for quicker and more effective treatment. One or two intravenous H_2O_2 treatments will usually suffice.

Peptic Ulcer Is Catching

The very idea that an ulcer might be contagious would have been preposterous a few years ago, but we now know that it's possible. It's also possible that you got it from something you ate or drank. If you are an "old-timer" with my newsletter, you heard about this discovery in these pages three years ago (long before medical students were being taught about it).

The culprit is a bacterium called Helicobacter pylori which likes to set up housekeeping in the stomach and the duodenum, the area that joins the stomach to the small intestine. It's choosey about its neighborhood and won't live in the small or large intestine — probably a racial thing. (Would *you* want to live with billions of E coli bacteria?) H pylori has a spiral shape and a screw-like motion that enables it to burrow into the mucous gel of the stomach and set up residence on the stomach lining. The body cannot throw off the invader, so you have it for life if it's not treated.

The treatment recommended today by the experts is a trial of bismuth subsalicylate (Pepto-Bismol) which, if you care, is approved by the FDA for ulcer therapy. If this doesn't work — and it only works about 25 percent of the time — then the antibiotic metronidazole (Flagyl) is added to the program. The doctors using this mode of therapy admit that they don't know if the combined treatment, which is effective about 80 percent of the time, is due to killing the H pylori bacteria or due to some curative effect on the stomach lining. (I recommend trying some cabbage juice for the pain. It might just surprise you.)

If the infectious origin of peptic ulcer is proven, and it's not totally settled at this time, it will have a tremendous impact on medical thinking regarding many presently puzzling diseases. Is rheumatoid arthritis an infection? What about multiple sclerosis, arteriosclerosis, and even schizophrenia? Karl Rosenow, one of the finest medical minds of the mid-20th century, presented evidence 50 years ago that rheumatoid arthritis is indeed an infectious process. He was ignored, of course.

Dr. Richard A. Root, professor of medicine at the University of California, San Francisco, remarked "I think that infectious agents may be important in many diseases in which they were once thought to play no role."

The lining of the stomach has always been one of those mysterious areas of medicine that makes us marvel at how smart the Architect of the Universe really is. (I'd like to hear the evolutionists explain how the stomach "learned" not to devour itself.) A remarkable balancing act goes on in the mucosa, or lining, of the stomach and duodenum. A mucous is secreted to protect the deeper tissues from the harmful effects of acid, which is also produced by the stomach. Most of the acid (and pepsin) is neutralized at the surface, but acid that does penetrate is neutralized by bicarbonate, which is produced by stomach cells. It's a very delicate balancing act between producing acid and then producing mucous, bicarbonate, and prostaglandins to protect itself.

Prostaglandins play a role in this protective mechanism, but how they do this is not understood. Scientists have demonstrated that *mild* irritants can protect the stomach lining from the corrosive effects of *strong* irritants without the presence of prostaglandins.

It is conventional wisdom that excess acid is responsible for the formation of peptic ulcer, but acid, a normal constituent of gastric juice, is inadequate to produce a peptic ulcer. *Most persons with duodenal ulcer have normal levels of acid secretion.* As in most areas of medicine, the more we learn about some disease process, the more there is to learn.[14]

Action to Take

1. This is a weird situation in that we don't have any idea how the disease is contracted. If it were caught through kissing, then we all would have it, or at least most of us. To be on the safe side, don't kiss anyone with active ulcer disease and use hydrogen peroxide to wipe cooking utensils and other things that the infected person handles.

2. The enthusiasts for H$_2$O$_2$ by mouth say it will cure everything from arthritis to old age — will it cure the ulcer infection? *I'm not recommending it;* I just thought I would mention it. If you try this, do not use more than 20 drops of H$_2$O$_2$ per glass of water.

Chapter 8

Some Impressive Case Histories

(Arranged alphabetically for easy reference.)

Arthritis

Both Mr. and Mrs. Anderson took H_2O_2 orally. Mr. Anderson, a severe arthritic, was "having a hard time moving. It has helped me tremendously." He took the peroxide daily for nine months and improved so dramatically that he decided to see how he would do without it. "As far as I can tell," Mrs. Anderson said, "he seems to have a permanent cure." It's important to note that arthritis comes and goes. Only time will tell if Mr. Anderson is really cured. See Mrs. Anderson's story under *Varicose Veins*.

Cancer

Another doctor horror story. Maybe you're getting used to them. I don't think I ever will lose my sense of outrage when I hear these cases; at least, I hope not.

Dennis Holder is from a little town in Canada called Amherstberg. He is a pleasant, nonaggressive fellow who sounds like he's from Maine-complete with the *aye?* at the end of a sentence in place of just a question mark.

He was devastated to find out that he had cancer of the lung. He had lost the other lung as a child. He was having recurrent lung collapse (called pneumothorax), so the lung was partially surgically removed. There's no doubt that it will never collapse again. There is little left to collapse.

But now there is cancer in the remaining lung. Not much to work with. His doctors said that there was nothing to be done. Holder was in terrible pain, only partially relieved by pain medication. He had to quit his job at the hog farm. He told his doctor that he was going to try hydrogen peroxide therapy. The way the doctor reacted, you would have thought he had said, "I'm going to kill myself."

The rejection could not have been more complete. He demanded that Holder return all medication, *including the medication for pain*. He refused to give him copies of any lab work or X-ray reports. He said that he wasn't taking any chances of a lawsuit. (Seems to me he's asking for it.)

Dennis Holder started taking oral H_2O_2 and quickly regained his lost weight and strength. His pain is now minimal, and he is looking for a job.

He then asked a *friend* whether he thought he should take some intravenous peroxide. The friend said he didn't think it necessary. Some friend.

As I have often said, people make momentous decisions based on the opinions of people with absolutely no medical training. But the way doctors behave, I guess you can't blame them. I urged Mr. Holder to seek out a doctor who would evaluate him for intravenous H_2O_2 therapy. His cancer was diagnosed only six months ago. The intravenous peroxide may prolong his life. I haven't heard from him since, but if he didn't take my advice, he is probably dead.

* * *

John O. Boxall, M.D., of Napa, Idaho, reports an interesting case of a cancer patient who lived 15 months beyond the longest estimate by all of the physicians involved. The patient was a 72-year-old Caucasian male with complaints of severe pain in the feet, and especially the right toe, with weight loss from 150 pounds to 109 pounds, shortness of breath, which had been present for about five years, and hypertension. The patient was on a number of medications, including Darvocet, Hydrocortisone, Tenex,

Lorezapan, and Trental. He had also been on Procardia, which depressed him so he discontinued it.

About three and one-half years before going to see Dr. Boxall, he was told he had emphysema, so he ceased smoking. Five years prior to this, he had his left lower lobe of his lung removed for adenocarcinoma.

At this time, he began to have mini-strokes (TIA's), and he was also found to have an abdominal aortic aneurysm (a swelling of the large artery leaving the heart and going to the abdomen).

He was hospitalized in December 1986 and was found to have a metastatic cancer at his left adrenal gland. His lung cancer was not cured, as this was a growth of the lung cancer which had formed in the adrenal gland.

Because of all these complications: spread of his cancer, hypertension, probably carotid artery disease and the aortic aneurysm, he was told by his doctors that nothing else could be done. He was sent home on one aspirin per day and some cardiac drugs.

In summary, what we have is a dying man who has come to Dr. Boxall for help. Dr. Boxall saw him on May 15, 1987. He was emaciated; he had a blood pressure of 180/100; he had the aforementioned abdominal aneurysm in his aorta, a minimal and restrictive breathing capacity, with cyanosis (blueness) of the toes and a large mass which was palpable in the left upper quadrant of the abdomen (the cancer) — a hopeless case.

At this time his creatinine (kidney test) was 1.7. Normal is 1.0.

Because of the seriousness of the case, Dr. Boxall gave the patient two hydrogen peroxide intravenous treatments on the first day, whereas usually one is given every other day. The patient noticed slight improvement immediately in his general well being. He also received treatment on May 20 and May 22. By May 26, the color of his feet had much improved, but he continued to have pain. Dr. Boxall continued the hydrogen peroxide infusions.

On May 11, a creatinine test was done and found to

be 1.2, which is within the upper limits of the normal range. BUN, another kidney test, had fallen from 55 to 43, a significant improvement.

Because of the patient's severe arterial disease, Dr. Boxall also gave him chelation therapy to improve his circulation.

After three months of treatment, 17 peroxide treatments and nine chelation treatments, the patient was clinically improved, feeling well, but he had not gained any weight. Despite the urging of Dr. Boxall to continue his treatment, regardless of ability to pay, the patient did not continue treatments and was not seen again until five months later, May 16, 1988.

The patient had stopped taking his vitamin E, which Dr. Boxall encouraged him to take again. From this visit and for the next five months, the patient received 13 hydrogen peroxide treatments and four chelation infusions, which was less than Dr. Boxall wanted but was all that the patient felt he could afford. The patient died about one month after his last treatment. He had received from May 15, 1987 to October 19, 1988 a total of 46 hydrogen peroxide treatments and 23 chelation infusions. The interesting thing about his case was, in spite of his multiple problems and hopeless prognosis, he lived 15 months beyond the longest estimate of any of his doctors.

***

Patient D.P. was a personal friend, as well as a patient. At about 11:45 p.m. on April Fools Day, 1989, his sister called me, almost hysterical, and stated that she found her brother collapsed in the bathroom, cold, clammy, unconscious and quite white in appearance.

The first thing a doctor thinks of in this situation is a massive bleeding episode from something in his intestinal tract. I instructed her to call the ambulance service immediately and have him taken to the hospital, informing them that his doctor's diagnosis was bleeding peptic ulcer with hemorrhagic shock.

The hospital staff agreed with my diagnosis and gave

D.P. two units of blood immediately. His hemoglobin was 12 grams and, in my opinion, the blood should not have been given because of the danger of AIDS. Unless the hemoglobin is below eight grams, blood is not warranted. Fortunately, tests done after he left the hospital were all negative for AIDS and AIDS-related diseases. His blood will be checked every three months for at least two years.

Subsequent tests in the hospital, including endoscopic examination of his stomach and CAT scan, showed him to have a mass, which turned out to be a large-celled lymphoma in the top part of his stomach and taking up over one-third of the stomach area. The mass was about the size of a grapefruit.

Against my advice, the patient started on chemotherapy 12 days after leaving the hospital. He continued to take hydrogen peroxide intravenously on a daily basis at first, and then at least three times a week. The peroxide treatment was started before chemotherapy, was continued during, and then also continued after he stopped his chemotherapy.

He noted that he had absolutely no side effects from the chemotherapy when he was also being treated with the hydrogen peroxide. D.P. said, "When you would leave town, I would always have trouble with the chemotherapy with nausea, vomiting and very severe depression." His doctors, he said, were puzzled that he had so little in the way of side effects from most of the treatment. D.P. said he also felt extremely fatigued and spent a great deal of time in bed when he would take the chemotherapy treatment without having had the peroxide.

D.P. lost his hair, as always happens with chemotherapy, and his toenails turned purplish and dropped off. These were the only physical signs of the toxicity of the chemotherapy that he noticed during the entire treatment.

Seven weeks after the first CAT scan another was done and, much to the amazement of his physicians, the tumor mass had completely resolved. There was absolutely no evidence of cancer being present. Granted, the patient was on chemotherapy, but I think any qualified doctor would admit that this was a truly remarkable result. D.P. told his

doctors that he had been taking peroxide and photoluminescence, and they replied, "Well, perhaps it's a result of
both his therapy and ours."

Four-and-a-half months later, in late August or early
September, D.P. had a repeat CAT scan, and again everything was completely normal with no evidence of any tumor.

D.P. lost 26 pounds in the hospital. By October of
1989, he had gained back all of that weight and put on
some additional pounds. He feels vigorous and healthy
and now is more concerned about keeping his weight
down than keeping it up. Parenthetically, it should be
noted that his chemotherapy injections cost him over
$6,000 per month. These injections cost him over $1,000
each. One of them cost almost $2,000. These so-called
chemotherapeutic drugs are all listed by the FDA as experimental, yet the patients are charged these atrocious
fees. If this isn't the biggest rip-off in medicine, it certainly
has got to be close.

Along with his peroxide treatments, D.P. also received
photoluminescence therapy on a daily basis. Both therapies should be given for maximum results in treating cancer.
A series of cases needs to be done with peroxide alone, photoluminescence alone, and the combination of the two to
determine the relative effectiveness of the two therapies.
Photoluminescence, the subject of another book,[1] consists of drawing a small amount of blood from the patient,
exposing it to a certain frequency of ultra-violet light, which
activates the blood, then injecting it back into the patient,
either intravenously or into the muscle. You will see in the
chapter on our AIDS clinic in Africa that the combined
therapies are showing quite remarkable results in AIDS.

An additional note on patient D.P. He continues to
thrive and work full-time, although he is in his late 60s,
and shows no evidence whatsoever at this time of ever having had cancer.

* * *

H.J. Hoegerman, M.D., of Santa Barbara, California
reports a rare case of blood cancer.

The patient, E.M., was a 68-year-old Hispanic female, first seen in August 1988. She complained of extreme fatigue and that every bone in her body felt tired. She had nausea and loss of appetite. Her vision was so poor that, without her glasses, she could not distinguish one person from another. She was brought in with the help of her daughter. The daughter stated that she spent her time in her home resting, being too weak to go out.

Her laboratory report showed an unusual picture, with anemia and nucleated red blood cells. This is very unusual in that human red blood cells do not usually have a nucleus, when taken from peripheral blood. Her hemoglobin was 9.8 grams (normal is 12 to 14 grams).

Because of the abnormal blood picture in this obviously very ill patient, a hematology and oncology consult was obtained. The report, which included a bone marrow study, concluded with a diagnosis of "myelodysplastic syndrome with predominant erythroid abnormality and a primary refractory anemia." This is a very serious disease, and, based on the blood picture, the patient was given a median survival time of one year.

Due to the poor prognosis and lack of any conventional or encouraging therapy, the patient was begun on a course of intravenous H_2O_2, alternating with intravenous megadoses of ascorbic acid (vitamin C), in a dosage of 25 grams. The routine was intravenous hydrogen peroxide on Mondays and Thursdays and intravenous Vitamin C on Tuesdays and Fridays. The treatments were begun on August 15, 1988, and on September 1, 1988, just 16 days later, after receiving five infusions of hydrogen peroxide and five infusions of Vitamin C, the patient was very much improved.

Dr. Hoegerman's notes on her chart in September read as follows: "Patient feels 50 percent better; she is no longer sleepy or tired; the nausea has stopped, better appetite and better eating. Her eyesight is very much improved. Vision is so dramatically improved that she came to the office unaware that she was not wearing her glasses. Prior to this, without her glasses, she could not distinguish one person from another; they were only large objects...."

Treatments were continued, and on September 12, 1988, the patient stated that she felt wonderful, much more energy, etc. At this time, she was working in her garden and going shopping. As of October 3, 1988, her treatments were reduced to once a week. This routine was continued until December 22, 1988, when lack of suitable veins prevented further intravenous therapy. She was then continued on oral supplements, which consisted of multiple vitamins and minerals, coenzyme Q10, vitamin E and vitamin C. She was last seen on February 6, 1989, at which time she moved to Mexico. She was feeling well and had maintained her improvement.

It is interesting to note that her blood picture also sustained dramatic improvement. These results are listed below, and, although you may not be medically trained, you can easily see the remarkable degree of improvement:

	8/15/88	12/22/88
Anisocytosis	4	0
Poikilocytosis	4+	0
Polychromasia	3+	0
Basophilic stippling	2+	1+
Ovalocytes	2+	1+
Tear Drop Cells	2+	1+
Target Cells	3+	occasional
Large Platelets	3+	0
Schistocytes	2+	0
Acanthocytes	1+	0

And most striking of all, the nucleated red blood cells had completely disappeared.

Dr. Hoegerman also reports, in addition to these rather remarkable cases: "I have seen several cases of bronchitis and pneumonia that were unresponsive to conventional antibiotic therapy which have improved within hours of IV hydrogen peroxide therapy."

Kingsley Medical Center
William J. Mauer, D.O.
Osteopathic Physician and Surgeon
3401 North Kennicott Avenue
Arlington Heights, IL 60004

SUMMARY

PATIENT: Charles E. Woodward   #6969 DATE: 11/28/89
PHYSICIAN: William J. Mauer, D.O.   1st VISIT 11/28/86

1. *History* 75-year-old male almost completely debilitated, barely able to get into the clinic, has undergone chemotherapy and radiation and refused any further treatment, having been diagnosed with bone cancer. The patient understood that we do not treat cancer, but merely try to enhance the immune system and he was willing to sign a release to this effect. His family was advised that he would do well if he managed to survive 4 to 6 weeks.

2. *Initial Complaint* Complete fatigue and exhaustion with digestive problems; unable to eat; a lot of stomach pain.

3. *Results of Diagnostic Testing* Showed a LASA [a cancer marker] of 35.5, Hemoglobin of 9.7, Hematocrit of 28.4 with RBC's of 3.14 and ESR at 140 plus, Serum Ferratin of 200 and Bone Imaging equivalent to that of an average 83-year-old male. [All of these lab results are abnormal.]

4. *Diagnosis* Metastatic cancer to bone, extreme immunodeficiency and anemia.

5. *Treatment Course* Began with multiple vitamin infusions; he had *14*, which seemed to be very beneficial, but he still was having a lot of stomach pain, and, as a result, had no particular interest in eating. At eight weeks, his LASA had gone down to 30.9, and on 1/26/87, it was decided to give him Chelox. After one treatment, the pain in his stomach completely disappeared. Currently, the patient has had 35 Chelox treatments and 30 chelations of EDTA. *[Chelox is a combination of chelation and H_2O_2 infusions.]*

6. *Patient's Condition Upon Completion of Treatment* Patient was able to resume driving and doing his daily activities without assistance, his attitude is good and his general health is greatly improved with the most recent LASA being 20.1 [approaching normal] on 8/23/89. His Hemoglobin was 12.5, Hematocrit was 36.8 - a very impressive improvement.

7. *Recommendations and Instructions to Patient and Date of Next Clinic Visit* The patient has been advised to have monthly IV's and supplemental injections for his anemia and his immune system.

Skin Cancer

Father Bennett (not his real name — "I have to be circumspect," he said.) is a Catholic priest. He developed skin cancer on his face. "Time after time I had to have the doctor remove it," he said. He took hydrogen peroxide by mouth the next time it returned and, to the doctor's amazement, it disappeared without further treatment.

"That's very strange," the doctor remarked. The priest smiled and agreed. Father Bennett now recommends peroxide therapy to his flock.

Mystery Illness

Steve Braun restores precious fabrics and rugs for the rich and famous. At the age of 34, he went into a mental tailspin. He had severe mood swings and such severe disorientation that he would be driving in Dallas and forget where he was going, and even where he was lost in his own home town.

Steve also had some type of elbow inflammation and wrist soreness. He was finding it difficult to write and work on the carpets.

We'll never know what caused Steve Braun's mysterious illness. Candidiasis gets blamed for just about everything these days (but Ebstein-Barr is gaining fast). Hypoglycemia, the diagnosis of the 60's, seems to be losing popularity.

Now, don't get me wrong. Any or all of these maladies could be responsible for Steve's condition. The only pop diagnosis we can be sure that he doesn't have is premenstrual syndrome. But we do know what cured Stephen, and that's good old H-two-O-two.

Steve started out with three drops of food grade (35 percent) peroxide in five ounces of cranberry juice, three times a day. He gradually increased to 80 drops a day. That is a lot of peroxide. Many people couldn't handle that high a dose, but Steve was determined to get well.

His pain was gone in a week. His head cleared within days, and he has remained completely symptom-free. After he became well, he began to reduce the dosage and now takes only 20 drops a week for maintenance. A dividend for Steve Braun was that his warts, a problem since childhood, cleared by painting them with 35 percent peroxide.

Candida (Yeast) and Chronic Fatigue Syndrome

Ebstein-Barr Virus (EBV) and candida yeast have been blamed for the chronic fatigue syndrome (CFS). This has never been proven, but Farr came up with some interesting confirmatory laboratory findings in patients complaining of CFS. Antibodies to both EBV and candida were significantly reduced, concurrent with an improvement in the patient's clinical condition, following treatment with peroxide. The patients complaining of fatigue had a significant improvement in energy and endurance with a reduction in complaints of fatigue. Farr noted this improvement may have been due to stimulation of oxidative enzymes and may not be related to a reduction in EBV antibodies in the blood. The patients with high levels of candida antibodies also noted a definite improvement with a reduction in their candida antibody titres. Mauer (see page 88) has had similar results.

H.J. Hoegerman, M.D., prefaced his report on the following case with this remark: "My experience to date with use of IV hydrogen peroxide has been limited by natural caution for a new and different therapy. However, even among this limited use, one case stands out because of its dramatic response."

This case was one of a white female, age 42, a college professor whom we can identify as Mrs. J.C. Mrs. J.C. was first seen in July of 1987. She was facing a new teaching position at a prestigious women's college, to start September of 1987. She was distraught because of the severity of her symptoms (fatigue, weakness, lethargy, fever and sluggish thought processes), which would preclude her from functioning in this new position.

Mrs. J.C.'s illness was of recent onset, two to three months, and had been unresponsive to conventional medical treatment (antibiotics and rest). She suffered low-grade fevers, mental lethargy, body fatigue and weakness. Her symptoms were of such degree that getting out of bed in the morning took all her willpower. This was in contrast to the alert, optimistic, fully-functioning individual that she was a few months prior to this illness.

Mrs. J.C. had read about Ebstein-Barr virus, which is sometimes associated with chronic fatigue syndrome, and wondered if this could be the cause of her symptoms. A complete physical exam was normal in all respects, as was her blood count, urinalysis, chemistries, etc. The blood, however, did show positive for Ebstein-Barr virus and candida, indicating a recent (reactivation of) chronic Ebstein-Barr virus infection. The candida, while positive, was of low titre.

The primary diagnosis of Ebstein-Barr virus was made with a secondary diagnosis of candidiasis. The patient was treated with large doses (35 grams) of IV ascorbic acid on three separate occasions, several days apart. For a day after her IV, she reported less fatigue, only to have it return in another day or two. However, her thought processes were generally improved. Although this degree of response was welcomed by the patient, it was obvious it would be inadequate for her to function properly in her new teaching position.

It was then suggested she could try IV hydrogen peroxide and, grasping at straws, she readily agreed. The first IV of 250 cc of five percent Dextrose and two cc of 15 percent Hydrogen Peroxide was administered, and the effect was immediate. The fatigue left within three hours, and her thought processes became clear and normal. Mrs. J.C. returned the following two days for similar infusions of hydrogen peroxide, hoping to sustain the remarkable improvement. She then left town for a two-week business trip to the east coast. When she returned, she reported that she continued to feel fine. She received one more IV of hydrogen peroxide and left for her new teaching position in good health and spirits.

Dr. Hoegerman reported: "I had continuing follow-up with this case. I can report that Mrs. J.C. has maintained her improved health status and has continued to function well in her teaching position as well as in life's daily activities."

***

Maggie G., age 35, got off to a rough start in life. She developed thrombocytopenic purpura at age six. A blood cell called a thrombocyte, or platelet, disappears from the blood in this condition. The blood becomes too thin, causing bleeding into the skin. This causes ugly purple blotches. If severe enough, the condition can be fatal.

Her spleen was removed because, for reasons not completely understood, this will often alleviate the condition. The operation did relieve her purpura, but other problems developed relative to her immune system.

She suffered from almost constant infections with unremitting fever. Her bones and joints ached continually. She developed diarrhea alternating with constipation, debilitating fatigue and severe food allergies. The spleen removal may have saved her life, but the price she has had to pay has far exceeded the hospital bill. After countless treatments with antibiotics, "I gave up on regular medicine," she said. She reasoned that the antibiotics had caused her to develop a generalized yeast problem. She eliminated sugar from her diet and took some colonic irrigations. She was helped considerably but felt the need for more intensive treatment of her candidiasis.

Fortunately, she was able to find an M.D. who understood and treated the yeast syndrome. Conventional therapies, such as nystatin and acidophilus, were of no avail. Because of her purpura history, the effective but dangerous drug, Nizoral, could not be used.

Maggie had heard of peroxide therapy. The renowned Dr. Carl Rosenow of the Mayo Clinic had treated her sister with peroxide for infection secondary to cystic fibrosis many years ago.

Her doctor, although open-minded, was afraid to treat her with hydrogen peroxide. But he agreed to

"watch her." Fair enough.
Within a month of taking peroxide orally, she im-

Kingsley Medical Center
William J. Mauer, D.O.
Osteopathic Physician and Surgeon
3401 North Kennicott Avenue
Arlington Heights, IL 60004

SUMMARY
PATIENT Jim H. Bayert #7512   DATE 12/7/87
PHYSICIAN: William J. Mauer, D.O.   1ST VISIT 12/7/87

1. *History* 39-year-old male was first seen on 12/7/87, with history of T and A operation in 1970 and Chemo-Papane procedure of the low back in 1981. He had no significant previous illnesses.

2. *Initial Complaint* Dizziness, fatigue, slow thinking, mood swings, craving for breads and chocolate, with depression, muscle aches, diarrhea, constant worries, anxiety, inside trembling, lack of concentration, vertigo and mental confusion.

3. *Results of Diagnostic Testing* On 12/7/87, revealed liver dysfunction, also Hypoglycemia with Hypoadrenocorticism. On 8/4/89, Anti-Candida blood test revealed an IGG of 239, IGA of 184, IGM of 118 [abnormal].

4. *Diagnosis* Functional Hypoglycemia with Hypoadrenocorticism and mild Hepatic Dysfunction. On 8/4/89, patient was also diagnosed as having Systemic Candida Albicans.

5. *Treatment Course* Originally was on a low carbohydrate, moderate fat, high protein diet, which satisfied innumerable complaints, but, as of 8/4/89, patient was still experiencing fatigue, vertigo, mental confusion, lack of concentration and mood swings. Patient was given a course of 10 treatments with H_2O_2 intravenously between 8/17189, and 10/30/89.

6. *Patient's Condition Upon Completion of Treatment* The fatigue, vertigo, mental confusion were completely gone, and the lack of concentration and mood swings were much better. Anti-Candida Test revealed an IGG of 36, IGA of 103 and IGM of 160 which is a marked improvement over the test that was done on the 4th of August.

7. *Recommendations and Instructions to Patient and Date of Next Clinic Visit* The patient was instructed to stay with his dietary changes, and it was decided to give him another 5 treatments with Hydrogen Peroxide to see if the Anti-Candida Test could be further improved.

proved *incredibly.* Her color went from ashen to pink. Her food and chemical allergies abated, and she had a marked increase in energy. By September of 1985, she was completely well and took on a demanding new job.

Maggie's case is very unusual in that after becoming well she developed a sore throat. I don't know what the explanation is — maybe too much of a good thing. Fortunately, this paradoxical reaction is uncommon. This should not be confused with the die-off phenomenon (Herxheimer reaction) or the Herring phenomenon. (But let's not get into that.)

* * *

Mrs. Dorothy I., age 54, was diagnosed as having candidiasis in *1984.* The diagnosis was made by dark field microscopy. This is a special microscope used to visualize yeast debris in the blood. The procedure is highly controversial but, in my opinion, has merit.

There is no question that the yeast can enter the bloodstream, but whether it is the yeast we are actually seeing under the microscope is another matter. I think it is. There are many ways to test for candidiasis. The blood can be tested for allergic reactivity to yeast. The stool can be examined microscopically for the yeast cells and, best of all, a careful history will often reveal a typical pattern of complaints consistent with the diagnosis.

After all that, if the diagnosis is uncertain, we recommend treatment anyway, because the therapy is not dangerous. If the patient gets better with a therapeutic trial of nystatin, desensitization injections (most important part of the treatment) or caprylic acid orally, then, in retrospect, you have a diagnosis.

Incidentally, Dorothy did well on peroxide.

* * *

Mrs. I. was one of those patients who simply didn't respond to any of these therapeutic modalities. Her symptoms, typical of candidiasis (extreme fatigue, depression, suicidal urges, food allergies, frequent colds, bronchitis and multiple skin problems), persisted.

This means that (1) she didn't have candidiasis or (2) it was resistant to all of the various treatments tried, including nystatin and caprylic acid.

She decided to try hydrogen peroxide. She slowly improved and lost most of her symptoms, including the depression and fatigue.

But the most interesting change in Mrs. I.'s case was her colon function (which she hadn't mentioned at the beginning of our discussion). She had diarrhea for 13 years without let up. About three months after starting the treatment she passed a *rubbery stool* which was a foot and a half long! She has had perfectly normal bowel movements since that disturbing episode.

Maybe she had candida and maybe she didn't, *but she got well.*

Depression (and Lupus)

As with most cases of lupus, Janet Johnson was initially diagnosed as having arthritis. She went to the doctor complaining of fever, being sore all over and too weak to get out of bed. She was put on Motrin and promptly developed a rash all over her body.

A medical center in Denver made the diagnosis of lupus erythematosus, and she was put on cortisone. She still takes cortisone, but oral H_2O_2 has enabled her to cut down from 10 mg of cortisone a day to two mg.

This is *extremely important,* because peroxide therapy enables doctors to use *much smaller doses of medication,* and thus may allow a drug to be effective without the toxic side-effects. As we mentioned on pages 79 and 80, this even applies to radiation therapy.

But just as important in this case was an unsolicited remark made by Janet. She said that her mental change was the most important part of her improvement. She had become morose, depressed, and irritable. If she quit the peroxide, her symptoms would return. It was so dramatic that her family members could tell when she was not taking her peroxide.

I have heard this story over and over again, and its importance cannot be overemphasized, because peroxide may prevent our country from being torn to shreds from AIDS-IBD.

AIDS-Induced Brain Disease is an insanity caused by the AIDS virus. *This is the worst form of AIDS* because, unfortunately, they may not die quickly. They can live for years in a dangerous demented state with no other signs of AIDS. Because of its effect on the mind, *maybe* H_2O_2 will prevent these people from running amok in our communities. I hope to God I'm right on this one.

Relief for Emphysema — An Impossible Dream?

Seeing John Houston, the great director, attempting to direct a new movie, *The Dead*, while *looking* like the dead, inspired me to report to you on that heretofore hopeless condition, emphysema.

There is nothing a doctor dreads more than seeing an emphysema patient walk or wheelchair into his office. They are usually thin (How can you eat, if you can't breathe?), blue in the face, gasping for air and thoroughly exhausted simply from trying to stay alive — a perpetually drowning patient.

We have little to offer these desperate people — drugs to dilate their bronchial tubes, oxygen and antibiotics when the inevitable infection occurs. That's it for allopathic therapy. Good physical therapy, with percussion to the chest wall and drainage exercises, is probably better than all the drugs.

How did these people get this way? Most of them have destroyed their lungs through cigarette smoking or a combination of smoking and some environmental factor such as coal dust, or factory fumes or radon exposure. It is interesting to note that studies have shown most pollutants, *in the absence of cigarette smoking*, are far less injurious to the lungs. Even asbestos causes little injury if the person is a nonsmoker. Smoking seems to be the catalyst for asbestos toxicity and also for radon toxicity.

We now have a treatment that offers an incredible, really astounding, degree of relief to emphysema victims. The first time I used intravenous hydrogen peroxide in one of these patients, I couldn't believe my eyes when he returned for a second dose three days later.

Mr. R. D. had terminal emphysema. He had arrived at that *last rite of passage* for the emphysema victim: a wheelchair with constant oxygen being delivered through his nose. His color was that of slate, and his lips were blue in spite of the oxygen — an obviously hopeless situation.

On his first visit to the Douglass Center he had just been released from the hospital after a bout of pneumonia. The next pneumonia attack was bound to get him, if heart failure didn't.

As with all of our patients with lung disease, Mr. R. D. began to cough 10 minutes after the treatment was started. After the third treatment, he had some difficulty breathing. We cut the volume of fluid in his infusion by half, and he has had no further reaction.

After four treatments, he discarded his wheelchair and discontinued the nasal oxygen. His face has become pink, and he sleeps flat in bed with no difficulty. He was having to sleep propped up because of inability to breathe. *This amount of improvement is unheard of in emphysema patients.* Another sign of his remarkable recovery was a return of appetite and a weight gain of eight pounds.

I am convinced that with peroxide therapy we finally have an effective treatment for these severely afflicted people. With the first treatment, the patient will often seem to get immediately worse, with violent coughing and production of copious amounts of phlegm. You can actually turn the coughing on and off by turning the infusion on and off.

Dr. Charles Farr, the pioneer in peroxide therapy in this country, calls it the *Alka-Seltzer effect.* The oxygen seems to bubble up between the membrane lining and the pus, thus propelling the pus upward. This stimulates coughing and removal of all the junk that has accumulated in the lungs. The end result is a very happy patient.

Chronic lung disease is not the only place for hydrogen peroxide by any means. But it is certainly one of the most dramatic uses for this safe and effective therapy.

Fracture With Nonunion

The condition in orthopedics known as *nonunion* is one of the most serious encountered in the field of bone injury. A fracture, often for reasons unknown but probably related to bad circulation, just doesn't heal. The ends of the fracture don't join together, leaving the patient with a serious disability; in essence, a permanent fracture. If this were to happen in one of the large bones of the leg or arm, it would be very debilitating and lead to permanent crippling. There is nothing that an orthopedist dreads more than a nonunion.

Patient R.T.T. was treated by Dr. Martin Dayton of Miami Beach for angina pectoris (chest pain of cardiac origin), uncontrolled diabetes and fatigue. The patient had a nonunion of an arm fracture, which was two years old.

After treatment with intravenous hydrogen peroxide, the chest pain completely disappeared, the diabetes came under control with the patient able to maintain a normal blood sugar and his energy level dramatically increased. Much to the surprise of everyone, including Dr. Dayton, the arm fracture completely healed.

"I thought it was a miracle," the patient said, "until I later discovered that similar healings have been known to occur with another oxygen therapy called hyperbaric oxygen." The patient was certainly correct, in that hyperbaric oxygen has been known to heal old fractures, but hydrogen peroxide can accomplish the same thing at much less cost and without any potential side effects. This is the first case of healing of a nonunion that we have encountered using H_2O_2, but, I suspect, there will be more reported following this remarkable case.

Lupus Erythematosus

Rose Medick, 43, tells her story better than I can: "I'm so glad you asked for my story. I feel like a balloon about to explode. I do diabetic and ostomy patient instruction at the hospital. I have wanted a doctor to whom I could talk that would understand, and not think I was crazy for feeling better on hydrogen peroxide.

"In 1978 we were building our home and I was in the sun a lot and was under the normal stress you have of building your first home. My joints hurt so badly. At night my shoulders and hips hurt when I slept. I was chilling every night-so cold-especially my nose and toes. I'd go to bed with piles of covers on and wake up at 3:00 a.m. so hot! I'd have a low grade temperature. I thought I was cold because the house was drafty and it didn't bother the kids because they were so active. I thought I woke up so hot because of all the covers. I was making excuses instead of admitting to myself that I was sick.

"During this time, I found that I would cry very easily. The world seemed so sad to me. Once when a sugar bowl was dropped and broken, I found myself reacting to it as if it was a major disaster. I would go to church and cry because it was too touching. I couldn't understand why my children were not as sensitive as I was.

"I hurt in every joint in my body, but not all the time. I was unable to run to the mail box which was a block from my house without being out of breath. I also noticed that I developed a red face while being in the sun. I also had sores in my mouth all the time. I would have a sore throat and cold, one right after another.

"In January 1979, my doctor told me my ANA Titre was 'speckled' and that I probably had lupus collagen vascular disease. He told me to take aspirin when I felt bad.

"I developed a chest pain on and off so I stopped a doctor in the hall at work and explained my fear of heart problems because of my family history of heart disease. He said it was probably pleurisy and the first step of treating Lupus was to take aspirin on a regular basis. When I took aspirin on a regular basis, I felt better. I later went from aspirin to Motrin.

"At the same time I also had frequency and urgency of urination. This was always worse during my period; in fact, all my symptoms were worse at that time. My doctor had me go to a urologist, and after doing a cystoscopic examination, he determined that I needed a bladder repair. I had so much faith in the doctor then. In March I had the repair done. I'm sure I didn't need it because within two weeks all of my symptoms returned.

"In June of 1984, I was told about hydrogen peroxide. I didn't believe it was for me then. In July 1984, Walter Grotz came through Nebraska from California and had a meeting in the basement of a community church in Ogallala, Nebraska. I attended and started taking 35 percent food grade hydrogen peroxide at that time. Two weeks later, I felt awful and was told I was supposed to, but in two more weeks I felt much better. I continued on 10 drops two times a day. That was all I could stand. The first thing I noticed was that I was happier. At this time I was on five or six, 600 mg Motrin a day. My chills stopped altogether. The arthritis localized to my middle finger and two joints in my legs, then that went away. I decreased my Motrin to 1,600 mg a day with no increase in pain or other symptoms.

"In November 1984, I woke up with terrible pain in the left kidney area and was sick all over. After drinking some water, I went to the bathroom and had pain on urinating. In the morning I went to the doctor and had blood in my urine, no infection. I feel that I passed a kidney stone. I went to the coffee shop and went to the bathroom again and there was a black speck in the water. I wish now I would have picked it up. I'm sure it was a stone.

"I increased my drops of hydrogen peroxide to 15 or 20 drops, two times a day. In March 1985, I developed a terrible pain, I almost felt like I did in November when I passed the stone, only the pain was from my naval to the pubic area and doubled me over. Later I had diarrhea. I went to the doctor, but I don't think he understood my problem, because it was over then. I just wanted a doctor to know how awful I felt in case it came back. I think he put something else on the record that I sent to the insurance company. The pain I felt was like something was tearing away my intestines.

"Later that year I decreased my Motrin again, with no chills or crying or hair loss. Every year in September, my hair would come out by the handful, and it would last most of the winter.

"I continued to feel good, almost too good, because I slacked off on taking the hydrogen peroxide during October, November, and December 1985. In December 1985, I felt a flare-up coming on and I started to chill in the evenings. I started having hair loss again and I became very tired and weak. I had some lab work done before I went back on the hydrogen peroxide faithfully again. My white count was 5,000. At this time I also had a serum complement reading of 44 — the normal is 150 to 250. This test is supposed to foretell a flare-up.

"I got the flu in February 1986, but was back to work in five days after a 2,500 WBC. In August, I cut my Motrin again. In September my WBC was 6,000; I was thrilled. I have also had less frequency and urgency of urination now. I went to Arizona in October, 1986, for a vacation and got a rash on my arms that was typical of a lupus rash. It was raised water blisters that itched, but didn't hurt. I ended up with two spots that didn't heal for a long time.

"I was 24 when I was diagnosed with lupus and I am now 42. I can sit Indian fashion now and no longer have pleurisy. Even though I feel better, I know the intravenous hydrogen peroxide would make me feel even better. I would not be afraid of taking it and I am even looking forward to taking it some time this summer.

"I very seldom go to bed before 11:00 p.m., and I'm up at 7:00 a.m. without needing to take naps. My worst time is still during my period, and even then it's not so bad. I go rock hunting with my husband, but I'm very careful with the sun. I feel I have improved the quality of my life in the last two-and-a-half years since first taking hydrogen peroxide. I am truly grateful for what H_2O_2 has done for me."

We have Rose's medical records, and they completely confirm her remarkable story.

* * *

Chris Springer, age 26, came as close to death from her lupus as you can and still be a whole human being.

She developed cerebritis, an inflammation and swelling of the brain, with convulsions and all of the symptoms characteristic of a major stroke. She had two serious bouts with nephritis, which almost took her away because of kidney failure. Doctors (including me) rarely diagnose lupus erythematosus at the first visit of the patient. Like multiple sclerosis, it can be subtle. Even what would be obvious to a specialist in lupus may be missed by the average doctor in practice.

But Chris had an early diagnosis because of two circumstances. First, she had the typical butterfly rash on her face. The rash, with open sores in her case, is distributed in a butterfly configuration across the eyes and nose. That sign should scream *lupus!* to any intelligent doctor.

Secondly, and probably more importantly, the dermatologist she went to see about the rash had a sister with lupus. (The closer a disease hits home, the smarter a doctor gets.)

A university specialist recommended Cytoxan for treatment. Chris is no dummy. She refused the Cytoxan, because, she said, "I didn't want to trade one disease for another." Cytoxan is similar to nitrogen mustard, the chemical warfare agent used to kill Americans on the battlefields of France in World War I. (Now, American doctors wage war with these terrible chemicals against patients.)

Cytoxan causes cancer and can be extremely damaging to the kidneys. If the patient has been on cortisone, a fatal infection may result from the use of Cytoxan. Chris was on cortisone (and still is), and she developed severe renal disease even though she wasn't on Cytoxan. The Cytoxan almost certainly would have killed her.

When her case was presented at the medical school, her doctor was severely criticized. "It's impossible that she could be so well now and have severe lupus. You did everything wrong. You didn't even put her on Cytoxan. She got better, if she really does have lupus, in spite of your grossly inadequate treatment." No mention was made by the patient or her doctor (who probably was unaware of it) that she was taking hydrogen peroxide. So much for university medical specialists.

Chris has had the worst possible lupus complications and by all odds should be dead. She continues to improve on oral peroxide.

Multiple Sclerosis

The following remarkable case of multiple sclerosis was reported by a colleague who wishes to remain anonymous:

"This is going to be a singular presentation of a case of multiple sclerosis which was, in our experience, most unusual. The treatment that we had administered was that of oxidative therapy (H_2O_2 intravenously).

"Multiple Sclerosis is a disease of unknown etiology or therapy. The article brought up the other day in the newspaper stating that there may have been established a viral etiology for multiple sclerosis should not be too surprising, in as much as that has been the concept for the past 20 or 30 years. To undertake a treatment using oxidative therapy should not otherwise be too unusual, since oxidative therapy is known to be anti-viral.

"The remarkable results in this particular case may be more than anti-viral in that the oxidative therapy itself may have had other attributes which led to the remarkable results that we're going to relate to you. In other words, there may have been other mechanisms, such as dramatic increases in interferon levels. There may be other factors with which we're not familiar at this time.

"This case is that of a white, 44-year-old male who was diagnosed with multiple sclerosis 14 years ago. During that period of time he has seen multiple doctors in multiple locations with varying degrees of minor success. As we know with multiple sclerosis, we have remissions and exacerbations, and that is what we found in the history of this gentleman.

"We also know that with multiple sclerosis, as time goes on, the exacerbations become more acute and the remissions less so. It becomes progressively more severe as time passes; that's why the 14-year period is so significant in this particular case. The significance of the remarkable results presented is multiplied by the total time involved or, looking at it another way, multiplied by a total lack of time involved in this particular case. Particular attention should be given to the frequency of therapy and the total time of therapy.

"Here again, we have a 44-year-old Caucasian male who presented himself to our clinic on May 16, 1988. At that time he required the assistance of his wife and our office staff just to get into the office for studies. Past history revealed that he was diagnosed with multiple sclerosis in 1975. At that time his presenting symptoms were:

Slurring of speech;

Loss of libido;

Leg incoordination;

Blurred vision.

"Though the signs and symptoms were mild at the onset, over the ensuing years both the pain and the in coordination became increasingly distressful.

"Following the diagnosis, the patient saw many physicians with limited success. Just prior to his visit to our office, he had returned from West Germany, where he was under the care of a very prominent physician. He had been under this physician's care for the past eight months.

"We saw the patient next in our clinic one week later, May 23, 1988. His complaint at that date was complete loss of mobility of his right leg. His other extremities were also very weak. His initial laboratory findings were reviewed with the patient and were really noncontributory. His only abnormalities that we were able to determine were his cholesterol at 240, HDL 32, and LDL 182. The physical examinations and laboratory findings were totally noncontributory. However, multiple sclerosis was reconfirmed on

May 23, and, with the patient's consent, we decided to begin a series of oxidative therapy treatments.

"The patient was given this I.V. treatment every two to three days for a total of 20 treatments. The important part to remember here is that this patient, after 14 years of no improvement, received 20 treatments in eight weeks.

"*June 6, 1988*:

The patient received his sixth therapy. The patient stated at that time that he felt much better. He ambulated a small amount on the weekend. He was able to walk up one full step, which was considered quite a feat by his family and himself.

"*June 9, 1988*:

Three days later, June 9, the seventh therapy. The patient stated he was feeling much stronger.

"*June 30, 1988*:

On June 30, the 14th therapy. The patient was now ambulating with the assistance of only a cane.

"*July 5, 1988*:

July 5, the 16th therapy. The patient was able to walk for four hours without sitting down. We later found out that this incident actually took place at a cocktail party. The story is most astounding.

"The last official therapy that he received was July 15, the twentieth therapy. This remarkable gentleman was seen in our clinic at that time and was last seen driving away in his red corvette convertible with the top down.

"This, in my almost 30 years of practice, is one of the most outstanding cases that I have ever been fortunate enough to deal with. It is because of that reason that I felt that it should be brought to the attention of this group.

"As I stated earlier, the total number of oxidative I.V. therapy treatments was 20. This was over only an eight-week period. This was also 14 years after having been diagnosed and having spent thousands and thousands of dollars on multiple treatments all over the world."

Q: "The other question I had is: Did you treat any other patients with multiple sclerosis?"

A. "Yes we have. Nobody with this type of response, and I have a comment that perhaps should be made at this point: This gentleman had just entered the wheelchair stage. When we saw him he had been in a wheelchair between one and two weeks. And I think that is very, very significant, because other people who have been in wheelchairs, say for two years, I really don't think you're going to get any kind of results anywhere like this. And, I think that before the wheelchair stage is where any good is going to be done, whether it is with oxidative therapy or any other kind of therapy."

Q. "And did they [other MS patients treated with oxidative therapy] generally improve, or was there just no change?"

A. "Well, as you probably are aware, with oxidative therapy my experience has been that you usually don't come in with a patient who has MS only. They'll come in with MS, plus lung diseases, plus whatever. It's rare to find a person with just one illness. When they start responding in other directions, they usually are very exuberant about their response. I would say that we had varying degrees of success, none of which matched this particular case."

* * *

Carol Nelson is a 32-year-old, loquacious Californian. She is a successful real estate appraiser in the Los Angeles area. She hasn't always been successful and, during high-school and college, she was convinced that she would be a failure in life. Carol had to *read out loud* in order to comprehend anything that was assigned to her. Can you imagine the determination it took to go through college that way? She wanted to be a doctor but realized her inability to concentrate made that an impossible goal.

At age 21, she developed multiple sclerosis. In 1984, Carol had to sell her house and stop working. She simply didn't have the strength to continue a normal life. In addition to her MS, she had severe food allergies, candida (yeast) allergy, and *severe PMS* (pre-menstrual syndrome).

Her MS started with numbness, and her left eye began

to deviate so that double vision became a problem. She also lost strength in her hands, and the bottom of her feet became numb.

Carol ran the usual gamut of doctors. She took a $28,000 loss on the sale of her home to pay medical bills, just to continue to live without going on welfare.

After spending $10,000 on doctors, with no results, she decided to take matters into her own hands and look for another approach to her problem. The doctors didn't believe that candidiasis existed and most of them didn't understand PMS. Her complaints of food allergy were met with a shrug of the shoulders.

"I decided not to take this lying down any longer. I meant this literally because it was obvious that I would be doing nothing *but* lying down if something positive wasn't done soon."

She searched for *three years* (now that's dedication) and finally came across "oxygen therapy." She doesn't remember where or how she heard of it, but "intuitively it made sense to me." (Women are like that.) She finally found a doctor in Los Angeles who was willing to try peroxide therapy.

Carol assumed that candida sensitivity was her major problem and was taking the peroxide therapy for that reason. She had no idea that the therapy would help her multiple sclerosis and hadn't really considered it. She had been told by the experts that she would have to live with the MS, and that it would only get worse.

About a month after starting treatments (approximately 12 infusions), Carol was combing her hair one evening after taking a shower. The comb touching her scalp caused a great deal of pain. She mentioned this to her mother, who replied, "Oh, you have always had a sensitive scalp like that. When you were a little girl I used to have a terrible time combing your hair." People are amazing in their differences and bodily peculiarities. Who would have thought that *return of scalp tenderness* would ever be recorded as the first sign of improvement in an MS case!

"A few weeks later," Carol relates, "my husband and I were fooling around in the living room, tickling each other. He tickled the bottom of my foot and I shrieked from the intensity of it. I asked him to do it again-I couldn't believe it. The bottom of my feet had been numb for years. We hugged each other and both cried with joy. We knew that I was going to conquer MS There was no doubt. We went to church that night and got on our knees to thank God for the miracle of hydrogen peroxide."

Carol improved so dramatically that she got the courage to experiment with her food allergies. "I am so allergic to wheat that if I eat a piece of wheat bread I am constipated for two days. I know it sounds strange, but that's the way my food allergy presents itself. I've had it long enough to know." (When the patient says something like that, the doctor had better take her seriously. It may not "make any sense" scientifically, but the patient is usually right.)

"So I sat down and ate a large bowl of shredded wheat, which is usually a killer for me. I had no problem with it, even though I had received only 14 treatments."

Carol's severe PMS was the next thing to go. The doctor who had been giving her progesterone injections was sent to jail (for heresy rather than malpractice, Carol remarked), so she had no source for the progesterone shots.

But, much to her surprise, her premenstrual syndrome ceased to be a problem. At first, she thought she must be pregnant, as that was the only time her PMS ever went away. Her period came the following week, however. She thought this was just a fluke, but, much to her joy (and her husband's), her PMS had completely cleared.

Her mind became so acute, she reported, that "I thought I was going over to the other side"-meaning her thoughts were coming so fast that she could hardly keep up with them.

An interesting observation in Carol's case is that her period will stop if she takes a treatment at that time.

"Within a half hour of starting the treatment, it's like turning off a faucet."

Carol's parting remark: "If I had gone with the program that the neurologist suggested, I would now be in a wheelchair wearing a diaper; I am now working full-time instead of being an invalid. I am completely well."

* * *

"Ten years ago I became paretic on the right side," said Betty West, age 39. "The doctors told me it was all in my head. I couldn't write or coordinate things with my right hand. Because my family doctor seemed more interested in the politics of medicine — he was big in the AMA- than he was in my case, I never went back to him after the diagnosis of 'neurosis.'

"After my condition was finally diagnosed as multiple sclerosis by a neurologist, I gave up doctors because, although he made the correct diagnosis, he didn't do a thing to help me.

"I went into holistic health in an effort to help myself. Without that change in my lifestyle and some spiritual improvement, I don't think I would have made it. The attitude of the people I worked around was incredible. They had me dead and buried. It was so depressing that I finally quit my job and went on disability."

Betty was dramatically improved after 25 treatments of H_2O_2 and had decided to go back to work. "Boy, are they going to be surprised when they see me," she exclaimed.

She found out about the treatment from the brother of a friend, who told her to drop everything and come to Los Angeles. He told her that his sister had been *completely cured* of MS through the use of hydrogen peroxide therapy. Betty left the next day.

Betty brought the formula back to northern California after 10 treatments and finally found a doctor courageous enough to continue her treatments. She lost a few weeks in her treatment schedule in the process of finding a doctor and noticed a definite deterioration during that brief period.

After only three treatments, she began to experience "spiritual enlightenment." It was like something was pulling cotton out of her head. "It really scared me at first. During the hiatus of treatment between Los Angeles and San Francisco this spiritual awareness left me. It came back to me with the resumption of the therapy. It has changed the direction of my life."

At the time of our interview, Betty was 90 percent improved and rapidly heading for 100 percent.

* * *

As with almost every case of multiple sclerosis, Mr. Ken Kellogg was not properly diagnosed for about five years after his symptoms started. The first symptom he noticed was a cold feeling in his right little finger. The coldness gradually spread to the entire hand. He applied a heating pad and burned himself attempting to warm his hand.

The next thing he noticed was "black spots" in his vision, and his eyeballs hurt. Next, he became wobbly. "I couldn't walk a straight line." As the disease worsened, his entire left side became paralyzed.

Although his hands felt cold, paradoxically he couldn't stand to be in a hot room. A temperature above 70 degrees Fahrenheit made him very uncomfortable.

After a few months of therapy with H_2O_2, his tremor went away and his intolerance to heat disappeared. His vision improved and he went back to work. He feels that he is about 75 percent of his former self — a goal he never expected to reach. He still has periodic attacks of fatigue, but he can continue to work in spite of them.

Pesticides

Clearing Pesticides from the Blood with Hydrogen Peroxide

An 83-year-old, white female had her house sprayed for termites (chlordane?) on October 16, 1986, and immediately fell ill with nausea, chest pain, abdominal pain, headache, dizziness, and extreme weakness. The symptoms would clear in a day or two after leaving the house, only to return within a few hours when she reentered the house. She made repeated attempts to return to the property but, after several months, when the symptoms were not clearing up, she abandoned her home.

On testing, this patient was revealed to have seven different chemical compounds in her blood, probably as a result of the termite spray. Of the seven, four of the compounds completely disappeared after six treatments, one weekly, with .0375 percent hydrogen peroxide intravenously. Two of the other compounds were greatly reduced in content, and only one showed a slight, insignificant rise in concentration.

This remarkable effect of clearing pesticides from the blood with peroxide is probably due to the increase in the metabolic rate caused by the hydrogen peroxide. This would decrease the time it takes the body to clear poisons from the serum.

Compound	Test Date 09/16/88	Test Date 12/07/88	Percent Tested Change
p'p'-DDT, Serum	1.1 mcg/1	ND* mcg/1	-10%
p'p'-DDE, Serum	11.8 mcg/1	8.7 mcg/1	-27%
Oxychlordane, Serum	0.9 mcg/1	0.6 mcg/1	-34%
Trans-Nonachlor	0.5 mcg/1	0.6 mcg/1	+17%
Heptachlor Epoxide	0.8 mcg/1	ND mcg/1	-38%
Hexachlorobenzene	1.3 mcg/1	ND mcg/1	-66%
beta-BHC, Serum	1.3 mcg/1	ND mcg/1	-66%

*None Detected

Sarcoidosis

Sarcoidosis with Pulmonary Involvement and Sarcoid Iritis

K. M., a 41-year-old, white female, developed malignant sarcoidosis. Sarcoid is a disease of unknown origin and today remains about as mysterious as it was 100 years ago. The word sarcoid is from the Greek, meaning flesh.

It is most apparent on the skin, where it forms skin nodules which were thought to be tubercular in origin. The nodules, which are just below the skin, cause a very unattractive appearance but, in the benign form, cause no further problems. The connective tissue, which forms around blood vessels, has a tubercular appearance. In its malignant form, the blood vessels become more involved; the patient has debilitating lung disease and may develop sarcoiditis, which leads to blindness.

When K. M. was first seen by Dr. Farr, she had increasing difficulty with breathing and had marked limitation of physical activity because of the weakness caused by her breathing problems. She had developed progressive, deteriorating sarcoiditis in her right eye over the previous 18 months. She was being treated with a cortisone preparation, which seemed to partially control the symptoms. But whenever she tried to taper off the steroids, the iritis became worse, thus making her a captive of cortisone. Her ophthalmologist had suggested that she would next have to go on Methotrexate, a highly toxic drug.

When first seen, K. M. was having a severe inflammatory reaction in both eyes and short, gasping, labored respiration. Her records contained a chest x-ray, taken in 1987, which showed marked involvement of the lungs with the sarcoid condition.

She was placed on a series of 20 treatments, one a week, with .0375 percent of hydrogen peroxide intravenously with the following results:

7/27/88 (two treatments) — shortness of breath significantly improved, and she "felt amazingly better."

8/10/88 (four treatments) — the shortness of breath was further improved, and her iritis was also improving.

9/28/88 (11 treatments) — patient had no further shortness of breath and only slight pain behind her right eye.

11/30/88 (20 treatments) — the eyes had completely cleared of sarcoiditis, and she had absolutely no respiratory problems.

2/1/89 — Her ophthalmologist reported, "No evidence of any active iritis."

This is a remarkable case in that it shows a complete clearing of a heretofore incurable disease.

Varicose Veins

Varicose veins had been a burden to Mrs. Anderson ever since her children were born. The peroxide treatment eliminated the pain of the varicosities, although the veins are still there. She had to take the steps to her second floor one at a time. After the therapy, she could ascend the steps perfectly naturally.

Mrs. Anderson reported that her "teeth cleared out" from the treatment. She had persistent pain around most of her teeth. This disappeared completely with H_2O_2 therapy. Mrs. Anderson mentioned as an aside that she uses one teaspoon of H_2O_2 to a gallon of raw milk, and it "keeps very nicely" for at least three weeks.

How Much? How Often?

As a general rule, the more acute the disease, the greater the amount of peroxide that will be needed. In acute influenza, for example, the patient might be placed on one treatment of 250 cc of solution with a concentration of .0375 percent hydrogen peroxide daily for five infusions, or less if the clinical response is achieved earlier. Occasionally, these patients will require a *booster* once or twice a week for an additional five to 10 treatments, especially in diseases that tend to become chronic, such as hepatitis.

In chronic conditions, the treatment may be given less often, but for longer periods of time. Examples of chronic illness in which long-term therapy might be employed would be chronic candidiasis, chronic lung disease, hardening of the arteries, chronic fatigue syndrome, or hepatitis. With this type of treatment, one might give 15 to 20 treatments, wait for 30 to 60 days, re-evaluate, and then, possibly, give another round of treatments. The following are examples from the Farr clinic of how particular diseases were treated, at what concentration, and at what frequency. If you are not into dosages, just read the "comment" at the end of each numbered paragraph. That will be reward enough. We don't expect you to treat yourself. ("He who treats himself, treats a fool" — I know from personal experience.)

1. Acute Herpes Zoster: 250 ml of 0.15 percent initially, then every two days, for a total of six treatments. *Comment:* Resolved completely in less than one week, with no residual.

2. Acute Influenza Syndrome: 250 ml of 0.15 percent initially and 500 ml of 0.15 percent the second day. Afebrile after second day, but additional treatment the third day of 250 ml of 0.15 percent. *Comment:* Resolution of all symptoms after the second day, with no residual.

3. Chronic Systcmic Candidiasis: 250 ml of 0.15 percent once a week for 10 treatments and then monthly follow-up for 10 months. *Comment:* Clinical response not observed until after the fourth treatment, then gradual improvement continued. Maintained on monthly treatments.

4. Severe COPD (chronic obstructive pulmonary disease): Initial 250 ml of 0.15 percent, which caused significant alveolar debridement and coughing up of copious amount of purulent material. Continued weekly infusions for six weeks, and by the end of the sixth treatment, the patient no longer was coughing. *Comment:* Pulmonary function improved and the patient returned to working full-time. Maintained on treatment according to patient's "feel the need," which recurs approximately every four to six weeks.

5. Acute Asthmatic Attack (12 year old girl): Attack onset 24 hours prior to treatment. *Comment:* Given 100 ml of 0.15 percent with complete resolution of the attack within six hours following the infusion. No follow-up treatment necessary.

6. Diabetes Mellitus Type II: 20-year history of diabetes, taking 30 units NPH insulin a.m. and p.m. After five treatments of 250 ml of 0.15 percent, insulin reduced to 30 units a.m. and 15 units p.m. Insulin reduced to 15 units a.m. only after three additional treatments because the patient was having symptoms of hypoglycemia. *Comment:* Discontinued all insulin after 10 treatments and given H_2O_2 on a monthly maintenance. Follow-up glucose tolerance test appears more normal. Will maintain on schedule according to fasting blood sugars in future.

7. Chronic Post-Herpetic Neuralgia: Post-herpetic neuralgia persisting one year following a severe herpes zoster infection on right anterior and lateral chest wall. Given 250 ml of 0.075 percent weekly for 10 weeks. *Comment:* Neuralgic pain substantially reduced after fifth treatment and completely gone after tenth treatment. Will follow up at three month intervals and re-treat as necessary.

8. Impending Cerebral Vascular Accident: 71-year-old man with sudden onset, two hours previously, of confusion, paralysis and weakness on left side of body and drooling and unable to speak distinctly. Initial blood pressure 190/100, pulse normal. Given 250 ml of 0.3 percent H_2O_2 started immediately. *Comment:* All symptoms significantly improved within 30 minutes and completely resolved after one hour. Patient did not return for follow-up evaluation, but was asymptomatic with blood pressure of 140/90 when he left the office.

Chapter 9

Peroxide Therapy, Africa, and AIDS

With the establishment of our African AIDS clinic, we are embarking on a new era in medicine. The despondent cry that *nothing works is* no longer true. The advent of bio-oxidative therapy, supplemented with photoluminescent therapy, means we now have weapons that will enable us to wage an effective holding action against the dreaded viral disease.

Although it is not claimed that bio-oxidative medicine is a cure for AIDS, we have seen cases in Africa that were in the last stages of the disease and have, after six weeks of treatment, had them go back to work and become useful, happy citizens again.

While the comparison is by no means perfect, the best way to conceive of what this combined therapy does is to think of it in terms like insulin for a diabetic. No one claims that insulin cures diabetes, but it enables the diabetic to lead a useful and happy life. Until such time as medicine starts using highly sophisticated electromagnetic and photo-biological medicine, the disease will not be cured. But, as in any war, you have to contain the enemy before you can beat him.

We left for Africa on July 25, 1989, via Frankfurt, Germany. Five days later, because of complications I won't bore you with, we arrived at our target country in Equatorial Africa.

The next three weeks proved to be an unforgettable experience-both good and bad. Perhaps, after we collect 5,000 or 10,000 cases in Africa, we can get American doctors and the American establishment to listen to us.

No one can predict the future, but we all like to try. I predict that 20 years from now, and perhaps sooner because of the AIDS epidemic, bio-oxidative medicine will be the mainstay in medicine and replace many of the toxic, useless drugs that are used today. There will always be a place for drugs, but I think almost everyone in the medical profession today admits that they are over-used and abused.

One of the obstacles to this treatment will be its very wide spectrum of therapeutic usefulness. The old adage is, "If it works for everything, it works for nothing." Generally speaking this is true; but in the case of bio-oxidative medicine, it is *not* true. As you've seen from the case histories, it is indeed a broad spectrum treatment, and there are very few places where it is not worth, at least initially, a try.

With God's help, and the help of our courageous and long-suffering friends in Africa, we will continue to move forward in this exciting, yet terrifying, new era of medicine versus disease.

* * *

Twenty-two-year-old Amina Nuh died recently. The Kenyan press is not free and information on AIDS is suppressed. The papers merely reported: "She died in the Aga Khan Hospital in Mombasa after a short illness and was buried on the same day in Muslim Cemetery."[1]

Uganda is an absolutely beautiful country, sitting astride the equator. The Ugandans, unlike the Kenyans, enjoy freedom of speech, freedom of religion and a lively, free and critical press. The devastation of the civil war which ousted the maniac, Idi Amin, is being rapidly repaired.

The people talk openly about AIDS and its devastation of the population. A photo accompanying an article by Uganda's Director of AIDS Control, Dr. Samuel Okware *(World Health Magazine)*, shows a grieving father praying by the graves of his seven children and grandchildren-all victims of AIDS.

Dr. Okware said, "A recent survey of 114 household contacts of 25 AIDS victims showed that only the sexual partners were infected." (How, then, are grandchildren catching AIDS?) He reported that tuberculosis (TB) and other diseases are increasing rapidly, and infant mortality is worsening. "Socially and economically, AIDS deaths on a large scale among the productive population will threaten agricultural production and development efforts ... political commitment is essential, *as is frankness about the disease.*"

Speaking on education, Dr. Okware said. "The slogan 'zero grazing' caught the public imagination — a folksy metaphor implying that people should not, like cattle, stray from their own pasture into another." Education is difficult, he noted, in remote communities with little access to television, radio or newspapers. The president — through his speeches, political organizations and church groups — is working to educate the people. "Many people find it hard to assimilate the bitter facts about AIDS transmission. We had to soften our campaign with light jokes and comic plays by theatre groups."

On condoms, he said: "We have to be cautious about advocating condom use until we fully understand local cultural practices and attitudes." Dr. Okware concluded on a sad note: "We are trying to improve palliative terminal care and general maintenance, including psychological and spiritual counseling with the help of church ministers ... admittedly, there is little that can be done for the Patients...."[2]

We pray (and hope that you will pray with us) that we can, through Peroxide/Photoluminescence therapy, help relieve the incredible suffering we found in Africa.

Whereas the AIDS-infected in the United States die of pneumonia, sarcoma and common infections such as tuberculosis, the African victim has many other ways to die-such as malaria, Chaga's disease, yellow fever and "slim disease" (malnutrition). Unlike many Americans, they suffer in silence, appreciating anything, expecting nothing. Most of the young people between the ages of three and 18 are orphans, the family remnants of a half-million deaths from the massacres of Obote and Amin. (They both live in opulence in Zambia and Saudi Arabia respectively.) So life has been very cruel to these young Ugandans. They are kind, gentle people. The injustice of it all could make you cry.

In many African countries, funerals take up a great deal of time. The festivities and ceremonies may take two full days. With the extensive dying from AIDS, you can imagine how much time is expended taking care of the dead, which must be added to the burden of caring for the near-dead. If this condition continues unabated, *there will be no one to grow the food.* The new infrastructure that the Ugandan people have so laboriously and patiently rebuilt — roads, hospitals, hotels, the telephone system, all in less than three years — will be for naught if the AIDS problem is not solved. As a Ugandan friend of mine put it,"Back to square zero." Many other African countries face the same fate.

Uganda was demolished by two homicidal maniacs. The Ugandans picked themselves up only to be cut down again, not by a homicidal maniac, but by a homicidal virus. It must be stopped. Uganda has had enough.

Death is an hourly occurrence in the bush of equatorial Africa. Cheetahs, working in pairs, attack and kill a wildebeest. The vultures then stand by awaiting their opportunity to clean up the remains. A lion attacks an aging hippo, but the hippo manages to escape, only to lie dying, half-submerged in a pond miles away from the attack. Large hyenas circle for the kill. And death is a daily occurrence in the cities. The people are not stalked by lions and cheetahs, but by bacteria, parasites and viruses. Mosquitoes are ubiquitous in equatorial Africa. The death toll from malaria and yellow fever is awesome. Expensive drugs, such as Chloroquine and Paludrine, are available, but who can afford them? Only treatments that cost pennies are feasible in tropical Africa. Bio-oxidative therapy and photoluminescence offer, for the first time in human history, life and health to millions of people suffering from these devastating diseases.

Although we know the treatment will be effective in a broad range of infectious diseases — the research is there; the results published in the old literature are irrefutable—we are nervous and apprehensive because of the awesome responsibility and the immense amount of confidence that is being placed in us by a few forward-thinking and courageous African doctors. If we are successful, and I am confident that we will be, equal credit must go to these dedicated physicians who have been willing to put their reputations on the line, face embarrassment and even economic and professional harm for entering a new frontier. We hope, with God's help and guidance, to bring about a therapeutic revolution in the third world with these life-giving therapies.

A grandiose and audacious objective? Yes, but we feel it is entirely within the realm of possibility with the weapons we have: Hydrogen peroxide intravenously (bio-oxidation) and ultra-violet light (photoluminescence).

Road to Maaka — *Highway of Death*

Running south from Kampala to the southern capital of the country, Masaka, is the major artery connecting Uganda with Rwanda and Tanzania. The trucks rumble by incessantly, delivering goods to the heartland of Africa from the major ports of Mombasa, Kenya and Dar es Salaam, Tanzania.

I remarked to Sula, our driver, how pretty the girls were, dressed in their long flowing dresses with large sashes hanging below the waist, looking very pretty and very African. I asked him if they dressed this way every day, and he said, "Yes, they do," and giggled slightly. I remarked how wonderful it was that the ladies all dressed so elegantly, even in spite of their poverty, and how proud he must be of the women of Uganda for maintaining their elegance under such grim circumstances. He again laughed nervously.

It dawned on me about an hour later that these were

not elegant Ugandan ladies maintaining the country's standard, but were simply truck stop prostitutes looking for customers. I, and probably you, envision a prostitute as wearing a short skirt that is about two sizes too small and a very tight blouse that bulges in the front. But that is not the Ugandan way. These truckers are known to stop for "tea breaks" two or three times a day, or even more, and to spend their evenings in the same fashion when not driving. This is the way that AIDS has been spread across Africa, having been imported from the Western World through the ports of Mombasa and Dar es Salaam. The first cases in Uganda were reported in the sad and suffering town of Masaka. It then spread back toward the other major city, Kampala, where 100 percent of the prostitutes are now infected. All of the prostitutes in Masaka are also infected. So the highway of death flourishes, and the truckers continue to ply their trade and their favorite hobby, which is enjoying the prostitutes, who are also plying *their* trade. In spite of the horrific AIDS epidemic, there seems to be no abatement in their business.

Even more shocking is to see Europeans having dinner with these diseased prostitutes, apparently oblivious, or indifferent, to the danger and the almost certain likelihood that they will be infected by having sex with them. It seems clear that Africa is being blamed unfairly for this epidemic, as it was undoubtedly brought to Africa from Europe by European businessmen, both black and white. Black African businessmen went to Europe, contracted AIDS, and brought it to their homeland. The white man also brought it from Europe, and now is taking it back. Although it is a well-kept secret, AIDS started in Africa more than a year *after* it was recognized in the United States.

I visited a Catholic hospital in Masaka and asked the nun in charge of AIDS patients how many cases there were in the area. She replied, "We have no idea." It seems that, through education, even the most backward bush family realizes that there is no cure for AIDS, and so they do not come to the hospital anymore. They don't even come in for testing, because they know the symptoms of

AIDS. When they contract AIDS, they die at home, and often will commit suicide, as will the wife or girlfriend soon thereafter. In fact, high tech suicide has come to Africa. The most popular mode of self-destruction is to remove the tiny battery from a digital watch and swallow it-death within 20 minutes. If you take two batteries, death within 10 minutes. No one knows, including the pathologists, how many people are taking the "time capsule," as I have dubbed it, because few autopsies are done. Diagnosis is often by supposition and by exclusion. There simply aren't the time, facilities, manpower or money to conduct autopsies on so many people.

When told by the nun that she didn't know how many AIDS cases there were, we turned to what we felt would be a more reliable source-the man on the street. Our driver, Sula, is close to the people. He told us they were burying between 10 and 20 people a day in Masaka. "All you have to do," he said, "is check the graveyards and see how many funerals they're having." As Ugandans do not believe in cremation, this is an accurate way of determining, at least, what the death rate is from AIDS. You should be very skeptical when someone says, "The AIDS epidemic is disappearing." The AIDS epidemic certainly is *not* disappearing in Africa — people are disappearing.

A young man, whose name is Kaggwa (which means in Luganda: *born by the side of the road*), said he did not have a girlfriend because he was too frightened. "I can't ask a girl if she has AIDS. How can you start a relationship like that?" Young Africans, far more than young Americans, are aware of the danger of AIDS.

We noted a number of casket-making shops along the road to Kampala. Caskets are one of the fastest selling items in equatorial Africa.

After arriving near the very heart of equatorial Africa, we spent two weeks in frustrating opulence at a tourist hotel, waiting to start our great treatment venture. It was worth the wait. They set us up in a private home with complete security and five bedrooms in which to treat our patients. The house is in a residential area about five miles from the center of town. It was frustrating to waste almost two weeks before getting underway, but the country is desperately short of supplies, and they simply do the best they can. The furniture they brought in was made at a factory the very day it was delivered.

The following case histories are from our AIDS clinic "somewhere in equatorial Africa." The government of this equatorial country wishes to keep the AIDS clinic a secret for many very good reasons. With the positive results that we are getting, we are sure the government will "come out of the closet" very soon, because they'll want the world to know of the incredible improvements we are getting with AIDS, and many other diseases.

Case Histories

N-, John (Bigo), age 34, male
(Our first Patient) CLASS IV

8/14/89
Occupation: writer, Temp:37.8, Pulse: 100
Weight: about 100 lbs., Height: 6'3"
Some spots in vision. Anorexia, sight of food causes nausea.

Pain at left lower abdominal quadrant (presenting symptom).

Bowels: diarrhea; Urine: o.k.

Cough; but not short of breath.

Lived in Paris: 1982-1986

First Symptoms: Fever, January 1987, and Anemia. Was well in two weeks.

Again sick in December 1987; chills for two weeks, then well again.

In July 1988, chills again. In August, violent fever, vomiting for four days, also diarrhea.

Diagnosis of AIDS made August 1988; Malaria and Typhoid diagnosed, also.

Continued weight loss.

January 1989— Diabetes diagnosed- was in acidosis. Was put on oral diabetic medication. Started gaining weight and felt well after the diabetes stabilized. Family history of diabetes; elder brother is diabetic.

Felt well until April 1989, when abdominal pain returned. Took an herb and got better. Took another herb which brought sugar to normal. Even ELISA returned negative, but Western Blot remained positive.

Early 1989 — Syphilis diagnosed. Treated with daily IM penicillin for two weeks- inadequate; treatment repeated, then o.k.

Got sick again in July (early). Now complains only of the abdominal pain, fever, and nausea with vomiting, diarrhea.

Treatment

8/14/89

8 p.m. H_2O_2 - I.V.

10 p.m. Photoluminescence

No nausea after treatment, no abdominal pain, pulse 100, depressed.

8/15/89

5 a.m. Photoluminescence

11 a.m. Photoluminescence

Nausea and vomiting returned. No abdominal pain.

4 p.m. Photoluminescence

5 p.m. Temp: 101 degrees F, (37.8C), Pulse: 104

No liver tenderness, kept fish dinner down.

8/16/89

9 a.m. H_2O_2 I.V.

10 a.m. Photoluminescence

No nausea.

2 p.m. I.V. Vitamins, Mg-1gm., K-20 meq.

Appetite improving. Asking for food. Cheerful.

Vomited once.

3 p.m. Photoluminescence
10 p.m. Photoluminescence

8/17/89
Pulse: 112, Temp: 37.7 degrees C.
8 a.m. Photoluminescence
9 a.m. I.V. Vitamins
10 a.m. I.V. H_2O_2
Power Out
4 p.m. Photoluminescence
10 p.m. Photoluminescence
Slight diarrhea

8/18/89
Retained breakfast
10 am. Photoluminescence
11 a.m. I.V. Vitamins.

Hot compress to sore arm. Now optimistic, "I'm going to get well."

Temp: 37.6 degrees C, Pulse: 104.

Room thoroughly cleaned, given bath, bedding washed.

3 p.m. Photoluminescence
10 p.m. Photoluminescence
Appetite good.

8/19/89
Ate good breakfast.
9:30 a.m. H_2O_2 I.V.
11 a.m. Photoluminescence
12 noon Nausea
3 p.m. Photoluminescence
Ate full dinner and retained it.
11 p.m. Photoluminescence

8/20/89
Severe diarrhea.
Starting oral H_2O_2 10 drops four times a day.
7 a.m. I.V. Vitamins/minerals
7 a.m. Photoluminescence
3 p.m. Photoluminescence
10 p.m. Photoluminescence

* * *

Our author-patient, Bigo N-, after five days of treatment, became dramatically more optimistic and cheerful and said, "I know I'm going to get well."

The next day, as often happens in clinical medicine, our hopes were dashed, as his diarrhea became much more severe. We felt this was due to a yeast infection in his intestinal tract, which is extremely common with AIDS patients in the tropics. I felt that something aggressive had to be done, or we were going to lose our patient from intestinal candidiasis. I made the decision to add oral hydrogen peroxide, three percent, to his regimen, and so began giving him 10 drops in a small amount of water as often as he could tolerate it. He received a dose of peroxide orally on the average of every two hours. "We are waiting anxiously for the result, and in the meantime, we are giving him intravenous fluids with minerals and vitamins to compensate for his intestinal fluid loss," (I recorded in my diary.) Two days later (8/22/89): The diarrhea had completely stopped.

8/21/89
Ate three eggs for breakfast.
9 a.m. Photoluminescence
3:30 p.m. Photoluminescence
4:30 p.m. H_2O_2, I.V. and by mouth
Severe diarrhea
9 p.m. I.V. Vitamins in 250 ml of fluid
10:30 p.m. Photoluminescence

Severe vomiting (caused by oral H_2O_2)

8/22/89
No diarrhea this a.m.; vein sclerosed, started new I.V.
8:30 a.m. Photoluminescence
3:00 p.m. Photoluminescence
10:00 p.m. Photoluminescence
500 ml D5W with vitamins; vomiting continues.

8/23/89
No diarrhea — H_2O_2 p.o., 8 drops three times a day.
9:00 a.m. Photoluminescence
10:00 a.m. H_2O_2 I.V.
Retained breakfast
500 ml D5W with vitamins
2:00 p.m. Photoluminescence
Temp: 38.0 degrees C, Pulse: 104
10:00 p.m. Photoluminescence

8/24/89
Ambulating without weakness around room. Taking balcony visits today.
9:00 a.m. Photoluminescence; ate breakfast.
H_2O_2 by mouth
I.V. Vitamins = Magnesium, one gm; 'C', 5 gm; B6, 100 mg, Folate, 2 mg

Follow-up Report From Dr. John B-:

"You must be wondering why I didn't start with the report on Bigo. *HE IS DEAD.* He remained as you left him for quite some time. His main problem was vomiting before eating, fever had gone, also the diarrhea. Somehow, Dr. A- and I decided to give him some 'appetizer.' (Cyproheptadine tabs, two of them). He became drowsy for the next two days! Couldn't eat. Third day recovered. His sister was about to return from the states so he decided to go back home. (His sister is a nurse.) Taken home on 9/6/89. On 9/18/89, I was called to see Bigo at his house. He was in a critical condition. It was reported to me by his sister (nurse) that he had had a pneumonia attack, which they were treating with ampicillin injection, 500 mgs every six hours. So I started him on I.V. H_2O_2, 2.4 cc in one litre D5W, to run for 12 hours. Repeat dose after four days. He was supposed to come for photoluminescence as soon as he felt better. DIED ON 9/22/89."

Bigo's case emphasizes the importance of not stopping therapy too soon. He died 16 days after stopping treatment.

W—, Sam, age 24, male CLASS IV
8/24/89
Occupation: Veterinary assistant
Chief Complaint: *Weakness in joints,* blurred vision.

Fever intermittently for one month. Disease started in February 1989 with diarrhea, sometimes bloody. Two months later, developed high-grade fever. Diarrhea severe: as often as 12 times a day.

History of sores and inflammation in mouth, anorexia; no vomiting. Had typhoid and HIV skin rash, now clearing. Some dysuria [pain on urination].

Lab:
Hemoglobin — 10 gm on 5/18/89
ESR — 110
WBC — 5300, left shift, toxic granulation (indicates possible infection)
Weidel — Negative
RBC — normocytic, normochromic
Social: Unmarried, never out of country. Source of AIDS unknown. Not pursued because of presence of family.

Physical History:
Grossly wasted. Losing hair. No fever, enlarged glands, thrush [fungus] or skin rash. Resp: Neg chest clear. Abdomen: No enlarged organs or tenderness. No neurological complaints. Weight Unknown — scale not available.

Plan:
I.V. H_2O_2 every other day

Oral H_2O_2 drops—10 (3 percent), three times per day
Photoluminescence three times per day

Follow-up Report from Dr. John B-:

"Complained of fever on and off for one month. Now gone. Weakness in joints — now ambulatory. Had lost a lot of weight: 9/5/89 weight was 85.8 lbs., 9/29/89 weight was 88.0 lbs. Had no appetite but now very good. Had diarrhea — now no diarrhea. Painful urination — now no pain. Blurring of vision — vision now clear. Patient wakes up at 8 a.m., takes a bath all by himself. Goes out in the morning sun. He sits up until 2 p.m. in the afternoon. Sometimes he comes downstairs for dinner with us! Completely ambulatory. I have taken photos. A remarkable recovery."

* * *

K-, Swaibu, age 48, male CLASS III

8/23/89

Occupation: Salesman

Started coughing four months ago, productive of white sputum — not foul-smelling. Some chest pain, evening fever; no night sweats. Began to lose his appetite and has had no solid food for two months. Two months ago developed diarrhea, profuse, watery. No blood noted.

Six days ago developed skin rash, which itched, and oral sores. Has had nystatin and ketoconazole treatment.

Polyuria times six per night.

Social History: Has two wives and 18 children. The firstborn is married, last-born is breast-feeding. He has been to Dubai several times and also to Kenya on business.

Physical History:
Pulse: 80
Afebrile, moderate wasting
No lymphadenopathy [enlarged glands]
Oral candidiasis present [fungus in the mouth]
Rash on arms and legs

Chest- clear (x-ray negative)
Heart- NSR
Plan:
HIV Test
Oral H_2O_2, 10 drops, three times a day
I.V. H_2O_2, 3 x per week.
Photoluminescence twice daily, first treatment at 11 am. today

Follow-up Report from Dr. John B-:

"He has a persistent cough (TB?). Diarrhea has stopped. Abdominal pain has stopped. He's now happier. And has become more involved with his business. As a result, his treatment has become irregular.

Weight: on 8/31/89 was 134 lbs.; On 9/9/89 was 136.5 lbs.

Appetite is good.

Patient still has itchy skin rash.

Treatment of Photoluminescence times 21 days, I.V. H_2O_2, oral H_2O_2, 8 drops four times a day. As I write, I haven't seen him for one week."

* * *

B-, Alex, age 27, male CLASS III

8/24/89

Occupation: Soldier

Fever intermittently for six months; diarrhea same. Some "pins and needles" sensation, six months.

First Symptoms: weakness, generalized skin rash, diarrhea, vomiting and abdominal pain. Some occasional anorexia.

Sore on penis for seven months (exam — chancre on shaft).

Mild, nonproductive cough. No chest pain.

Some fever intermittently in evenings.

Treatments for illness have been unsuccessful.

Social:

Wife died of AIDS in January of 1989 after a long illness

with diarrhea, "slim," and fever. One of their children, age 14 months, died similarly (presumably with AIDS) four months previously.

Physical History:
Slight wasting — only slight weight loss (8 lbs.)
Afebrile. Pulse — 72
Large, bilateral inguinal lymphadenopathy
Healed M-P rash
*ENT-*no thrush
Chest/Heart- Negative
Central Nervous System- WNL

Plan:
Photoluminescence treatment for three days per week or more;
Oral H_2O_2, drops 8-10, 3 times per day
Monitor weight (present weight unknown)

Treatment:
8/24/89
9 a.m. Photoluminescence
2 p.m. Photoluminescence
6 p.m. Photoluminescence
H_2O_2 by mouth, 3 times per day
Profuse watery diarrhea cleared after two doses of oral H_2O_2/Photoluminescence combination.

Follow-up Report From Dr. John B-:

"Fever on and off since June 1st — completely gone.
Diarrhea on and off — gone after a week of treatment.

Sore on the penis for seven months-now dried up and healed! Patient is very happy about it. Within four days the chancre started drying. Appetite improved. Weight on 9/1/89 was 112 lbs.; on 9/7/89 it was 119 lbs. Patient discharged in good condition. Still had the itchy skin rash. No other complaint. Reported back on 9/15/89 for blood check up."

* * *

K-, Francis, age 26, male CLASS VI

Poor historian

Was well until seven months ago, when he developed diarrhea, vomiting and oral sores.

He also developed a fever of high grade associated with rigors. Later, he developed diarrhea and vomiting with general weakness and oral sores. (Sister reports that he developed the skin rash before the onset of all these symptoms.) He was admitted and treated for Typhoid. He improved. Given Nystatin ointment for oral sores, chloramphenicol and Septra. Discharged and stayed home for six months.

In April this year, he developed soreness in the throat, continuing up to now. Has a cough productive of pus-like sputum with a foul smell. Has associated chest pain. History of diarrhea, but now has stopped. Hasn't eaten any solid food since June (two months).

Passes a pus-like discharge per urethra and has penile sores.

Treatment:

Nystatin, Davtrin, Nimorial — no improvement.

He is very confused. Not married. Soldier. Has three children, each with different mother. Eldest six years; youngest four years.

10/4/89: Sed rate 65; Hemoglobin-11.3 [abnormal]

1/23/89: Scant malaria parasites

7/25/89: Sputum for TB, none seen

WBC: 3600 [depressed white blood count]

6/7/89 - 6/14/89: Admitted at _____, diagnosis of "Pharyngitis," chest x-ray- normal.

8/16/89: 2:30 p.m.

Temp 100.4 degrees, Pulse 120, Respiration 52, shallow

Emaciated, febrile, hot skin. No adenopathy. No skin lesions.

Chest — shallow resp., hyperresonant to percussion.

Heart — tachycardia

Abdomen — no organomegaly or tenderness.

2:45 p.m. H_2O_2 I.V.
3:15 p.m. Photoluminescence
4:30 p.m. Photoluminescence
5:00 p.m. 10 million units aqueous penicillin I.V.
5:30 p.m. Photoluminescence
6:30 p.m. Photoluminescence
10:00 p.m. Photoluminescence
Patient appears terminal
1:00 a.m. Photoluminescence

8/17/89
5:00 a.m. H_2O_2 I.V.
5:30 a.m. Photoluminescence
6:00 a.m. Pulse- ?, Temp 101 degrees, Resp 50
7:10 Patient died.

* * *

O—, Anne, age 36, female CLASS I

8/22/89
Occupation: banking
Girlfriend of patient, Bigo N-, is asymptomatic.
Plan: Photoluminescence twice a day while living here; then as often as will come in for treatment. Minimum of three treatments per week.
Will give in the muscle because of small veins.
Treatment
8/23/89
Catheter in vein
Photoluminescence twice
8/24/89
Photoluminescence twice
Patient did not continue treatment.

* * *

My Reply to "Doctor John":
Dr. John B-
P.O. Box 9996
.., ..., Africa

Dear John:

Thank you very much for your report of 10/2/89.

I was upset and depressed to hear about Bigo's death. Please convey my sincerest sympathy and regrets to Dr. David and his family.

Bigo's death points out a very important and serious trend that may be developing in your bio-oxidative/photoluminescence practice. The patients, once they make a dramatic improvement, seem to be leaving the program, thinking that they don't need any further treatment. It seems to me we need to emphasize from the first day of therapy that they *must not* abandon the therapy simply because they are feeling so much better. They need to take two treatments a day until marked improvement is found, and then, perhaps, once a day for a few weeks, and then three times a week and so forth; but they should never take less than one treatment a week no matter how well they have done. Weekly treatment should be continued indefinitely, or until such time as the T-4 cell count can be done on a fairly routine basis in ___ and found to be normal.

I do hope they will soon provide you with some help, because, obviously, the program cannot grow if you are continuing to do all of this work by yourself. With the success that we have had, the program is bound to grow if it is allowed to. I don't think, quite frankly, that the secret can be kept much longer, simply because the results have been so good. The patients are going to talk about their excellent results, and there is no way in the world that it can be stopped.

The healing of Alex's seven-month chancre is nothing short of incredible. I hope the army will insist that he come back at least weekly for treatment, preferably three times a week and then tapering off, if that can be arranged. We certainly don't want to lose all of the wonderful gains that we have made with him.

I am also very pleased with the improvement of K. I'm afraid that he is going to slack off on his treatments because of his busy schedule. As you note, he hasn't been

back in a week. *This is a serious mistake,* and I think we need
to make every effort to convince these people that they
must taper off and not suddenly stop their treatments.
Otherwise, they will certainly regret it.

Concerning your question about the oral hydrogen
peroxide, remember that Bigo did not start to improve at
all until we gave him the oral peroxide to clear up his intestinal candidiasis. If a patient doesn't have oral thrush
or any intestinal symptoms, certainly I agree that the oral
peroxide is not necessary. But it is absolutely essential if
they have any intestinal symptoms whatsoever.

As you may recall, I felt very optimistic about Sam. I
just had a feeling, because of his youth, basically, that if he
stuck with the program he would have a good result. Certainly, that has proven to be true, and I am delighted.
Let's not let up on him and continue at least b.i.d. treatment as long as you feel he continues to need that frequency. Then, of course, we'll impress upon him the fact
that he must taper off so as not to lose the wonderful gains
that he has made. Even if he completely recovers, he
should take at least one peroxide a month and a photo
RX fortnightly.

I will see what I can do about getting some multiple vitamin injectable, multiple dose vials for you. Concerning
the peripheral neuropathy, I think it would be advisable
to try the 20 million units of Penicillin once, or even twice,
daily for about five days in these cases, because many of
these AIDS patients do have central nervous system disease that masquerades as other things, especially syphilis. I
do think it is worth a try. I sent a billion units of Penicillin
that I purchased in Nairobi to Dr. A-, and I believe that
you have some Penicillin there on hand.

Your modification of the IV hydrogen peroxide
sounds perfectly fine to me. One must adjust according to
what one has to work with.

As a mouthwash, I would recommend the full three
percent hydrogen peroxide, as long as the patient can tolerate it. It is certainly safe at that dilution for a mouth-

wash, although, of course, I would not recommend that they swallow it. If the mouth is too tender, then I would start out, as you suggest, with a half-strength solution and build up to three percent as soon as the patient can tolerate it.

It is perfectly o.k., when the power goes out, to simply put the blood in the refrigerator where it will at least stay cool, and instruct everyone to leave the refrigerator door shut as much as possible, so as to keep the blood cool. If the refrigerator stays cool, then I would say that the blood can be used for as long as 12 hours. When the power comes on, I would expose it to another full eight minutes in the machine.

John, I think often of our wonderful evenings out on the porch watching the beautiful African sunset while we enjoyed a little refreshment and talked about Africa and the African people. I learned more in those visits with you about the country and its people than I did from everybody else in Africa, with the possible exception, of course, of B-. It was a wonderful experience for me, and I feel very fortunate to have a colleague in Africa who has such a good feeling for his people and such a natural, as well as highly trained, talent for the medical profession. I am very lucky (and Africa is very lucky) to have you in this program, and our colleague was very wise to have chosen you for this important work.

Please convey my warm regards to our three colleagues in this project. They have handled the whole situation quite wisely, and soon the whole world is going to be looking at Africa and watching the miracles that are taking place there.

Again, thanks, John, for the excellent report; and I look forward to hearing from you again soon on these and other patients. These will all be included in the book I am writing. I know that you are working very, very hard, but in the long run it is certainly going to be of great benefit to you and, of course, to mankind. I wish I were there to work with you and, hopefully, one of these days, possibly, I can move there and be more personally involved. I am

very grateful to you for your hard work and sacrifice in
this great endeavor.

Your brother and colleague,

Bill

William Campbell Douglass, M.D.

Chapter 10

Some Questions and Answers

Q: I have been reading about products that are supposed to be an improvement over the taking of hydrogen peroxide by mouth. Do they have any advantage over hydrogen peroxide? — *E.J.W., Colorado*

A: I think all these "improved oxidation-enhancing" products are a waste of money and, if you are taking peroxide by mouth, you are just as well off with the drugstore variety. This is not meant to be a declamation or endorsement of peroxide by mouth, but just "shopping advice."

Q: Many people are plagued with moles and in searching through medical books there is little mention of the cause or the cure. Do you have any suggestions? — *M.B.F., Wisconsin*

A: A mole, also called a nevus, may have a number of causes. Most of them are benign, but are certainly not attractive. Before going to a surgeon to have a mole excised or burned off, try applying three percent hydrogen peroxide to the nevus with a cotton swab twice daily. You can get the H_2O_2 at your local drug or grocery store. As we get older our skin is subject to many strange blotches, stains, warts, and moles. I hate to say it, but these are signs of aging skin and, in my opinion, have nothing to do with sun exposure.

The exception to this is basal cell cancer, a locally growing form of cancer that is related to sun exposure over many years. These need excising. The problem is that you are not qualified to diagnose basal cell cancer or the more dangerous squamous cell cancer. So, if a lesion on your skin doesn't respond to the peroxide treatment within six weeks, I recommend that you see a dermatologist. He will *almost always* recommend an "excisional biopsy," which means: "We are going to biopsy it by completely removing it and then if it is malignant, it will be gone anyway and you will be cured."

This logic is a little hard for you to resist as you have no way of knowing whether the lesion has the appearance of cancer. I would ask him: "Doctor, do you think this thing looks at all suspicious? I mean, do you *really* think it is necessary to excise it? Would I be endangering my life if we waited?

Of course, if you want the "thing" off for cosmetic reasons, then go for it.

Q. My son has cystic fibrosis. Could he be helped with light therapy and hydrogen peroxide? — *D.W.A., California*

A. I have been asked, at one time or another, if the use of intravenous hydrogen peroxide and ultraviolet light (photox) will help almost every disease known to mankind. My answer, in most cases, is "I don't know." Unfortunately, I must give the same answer in this case. I would say that photox is probably ineffective for the basic disease of the pancreas. However, most patients with chronic diseases are subject to infections which photox will help, so the treatment might be useful for a better quality of life.

Q. On page 52, you mention that H_2O_2 therapy is good for hepatitis but you didn't say which kind: A, B, or C. Is it good for all three varieties? — *T.E., Saudi Arabia*

A. Yes, hydrogen peroxide therapy is good for all three types of hepatitis (inflammation of the liver).

Q. I'm interested in food-grade hydrogen peroxide. If peroxide is an oxidant, and we are supposed to take antioxidants, isn't there a conflict here? — *C.J., California.*

A. There is nothing foody about 35 percent hydrogen

peroxide. It is powerful stuff and I think it is dangerously misleading to call it food, or imply that it is safe to take as you would food. The implication is that it is purer than other grades of peroxide, but analysis has proven that this is not so. If you are going to take peroxide at all, I would simply buy the three percent chemical at your local drug store. It is very cheap and no more contaminated than the "food grade." If you take ten drops of that, twice a day, you will get very little in the way of contaminants. Remember, I am not recommending that you take it *at all* because I have no scientific basis for doing so.

Not that I don't get "unscientific" at times. My great-grandma Bell taught me a lot of unscientific medicine, but she dealt with natural remedies from the earth, not something from a chemical factory that you are told to drink.

Intravenous H_2O_2 in *extremely minute doses* is another matter. It is backed by excellent, exhaustive research. When the purveyors of peroxide "food" can come up with similar research proving effectiveness *and* safety of large doses of peroxide by mouth, then I will recommend it.

Q. We have a loved one who has Alzheimer's disease. Other than a low-fat diet, vitamin and mineral supplements, daily exercise, and EDTA chelation twice a week, can you suggest anything else? — *name withheld on request.*

A. Essentially, I have two more suggestions. First, make sure your loved one isn't suffering from hypothyroidism (see my article in the September 1994 *Second Opinion*). Second, oxygenation is very important in these neurological diseases. The chelation is fine, but I would add oxygenation in the form of I.V. peroxide therapy. Contact the International Oxidative Medicine Association (P.O. Box 891954, Oklahoma City, OK 73189, 405-478-4266) for a list of doctors competent in this field. The list is available for a $5 donation.

One more point in your letter deserves comment. I see no reason for restricting fats in the diet of a chronically ill person unless there are very compelling reasons. Animal

fat is nutritious and gives energy to the patient, no matter
what the age. *Vegetable* fat, especially the processed variety
found in junk foods, should be avoided. And remember
that cholesterol is *absolutely essential* for proper nerve function — a low cholesterol diet is the *wrong thing to do* in
these neurological conditions.

**Q. I was so impressed with your book on hydrogen
peroxide that I have started taking the 35 percent food
grade. Your book contains case after case of successful
cures, but in your recent *Second Opinion* you say you don't
recommend it — has Kessler gotten to you? — *R.D., Washington***

A. People always want black or white answers. But
even if you give them clear *alternatives*, where black or
white is not possible and you are attempting to be honest
with the reader, people will misinterpret what you say.

I use five pages in the book to explain the oral peroxide controversy. On page 36, I said: "I have good friends
who use oral H_2O_2 in their practice. I have good friends
who claim that it's dangerous to use it orally. All I can do is
present both sides and let you make up your own mind as
to whether it is safe."

In attempting to present the pros and cons on the
subject I have apparently made some people angry. People say they want to take more responsibility for their
health yet, when you give them two choices, they get nasty.
They want a clear "Go" or "No Go" answer. For ethical and
legal reasons, I simply cannot provide that in the case of
hydrogen peroxide taken by mouth. And, no, Kessler
hasn't gotten to me. I don't back down on my position because of pressure — not even to subscribers, much less a
vainglorious medical enforcer like Kessler.

On pages 37 and 38, I said (emphasis in the original):
"I don't think H_2O_2 is dangerous taken orally as long as
the recommended dose is not exceeded (ten drops of
three percent H_2O_2 three times a day). But *a caveat*: Dr.
Charles Farr, who probably knows the research literature
better than anyone, does not agree. *Recent research confirms*

Dr. Farr's doubts. Dr Farr says that further evidence exists that H_2O_2 should *not* be taken by mouth, especially when there is food in the stomach. If you do take H_2O_2 orally (and this is *not* a recommendation that you do so), take it on an empty stomach."

I report on a few cases where peroxide was used with apparent success when taken orally. I also, to keep the report as balanced as possible, report on a few cases where peroxide was clearly not successful. All the other reports, indeed "case after case," as R.D. says, involved the use of *intravenous* H_2O_2. Reread the book, R.D., and you will see that I have *not* endorsed peroxide by mouth and I have *never* endorsed the use of so-called food grade peroxide. When giving a dosage, I am merely trying to prevent people from killing themselves, as a friend of mine almost did with massive doses of "food grade" peroxide. Because it was labeled as food, he thought it must be safe — a logical, but erroneous, conclusion.

Q. You mentioned the use of H_2O_2 as nose drops to prevent bad breath from chronic sinus infection. But what concentration do you recommend — straight from the drug store undiluted? — *Dr. B.W., California*

A. My daughter, who is stronger than I, takes it straight from the bottle and snorts it. I tried that and I thought my sinuses were going to fall out in a smoking heap. I dilute the three percent drug store peroxide half and half with water and use five to ten drops (depending on whether I have cat breath or dog breath that particular day), once or twice daily.

Q. I was in excellent health until age 76, when I was diagnosed as having bronchial asthma and emphysema. I was put on Ventolin and Vanceril. After three years, I came down with polymyalgia rheumatica. I would like to get off the drugs and wondered if intravenous hydrogen peroxide might help. — *E.V.B., Connecticut.*

A. People don't usually develop bronchial asthma at the age of 76. I think your diagnosis is more likely to be

adult respiratory distress syndrome, ARDS. We don't
know what it is, just as we don't know what asthma is. Both
induce a spasm of the bronchial tubes, and we have a lot
to learn about both of these diseases.

Ventolin is a bronchial dilator and Vanceril is a form
of cortisone. Although there is nothing that I can find in
the literature that would indicate that you contracted polymyalgia rheumatica (PR) from these medications, one
cannot help but wonder if three years of these medications might have induced the condition. We know less
about PR than we do bronchial asthma or ARDS.

H_2O_2, being a broad spectrum therapy (i.e., a sup-
plier of oxygen to the tissues), may help in your case. It
may not, but I consider it worth a try. I suggest that you
contact the American College for the Advancement of
Medicine, 23121 Verdugo Drive, #204, Laguna Hills, CA
92653, 1-800-532-3688, and ask them for the name of a
doctor in your area that practices alternative medicine.

Once you've found such a doctor, ask him about
these possibilities and see if he can't give you a more precise diagnosis than you've had in the past. Such a doctor
should also be able to advise you specifically on peroxide
therapy.

**Q. Some are saying hydrogen peroxide is good as a
cancer cure. Is the hydrogen peroxide "cure" a cruel hoax
or is it helpful as a treatment for cancer?** — *N.V.W., Illinois*
A. Hydrogen peroxide is not a cure for cancer, either
by mouth or intravenously. It can be helpful in treatment
because cancer is "anerobic," i.e., grows without oxygen.
Hydrogen peroxide increases the oxygen content of the
tissues and thus may slow the growth of cancer. Hydrogen
peroxide combined with ultraviolet irradiation of the
blood shows great promise — we are working on it.

**Q: With regard to the use of hydrogen peroxide ther-
apy, if an improvement is achieved in treating a given disease, how long will it last? Can the therapy be used to treat
flu or pneumonia in place of an antibiotic? And finally,**

could peroxide therapy reduce the amount of drugs being taken for a given condition?

A: It's impossible to tell how long improvements from peroxide therapy will last. As with any therapy, it depends on the condition, the person, and a lot of unknown factors. You can't get a 50,000 mile, 5-year guarantee with any therapy. In any chronic condition, such as emphysema, therapy will undoubtedly have to be continued on an intermittent basis indefinitely.

H_2O_2 therapy is very effective on flu and pneumonia, especially if used in conjunction with ultraviolet blood irradiation (photoluminescence).

One of the major benefits of peroxide therapy is the elimination of the need for drugs. In fact, most or all drugs can be eliminated in the treatment of infectious diseases by using the combination of H_2O_2 and ultraviolet light therapy.

Q. I have been diagnosed with multiple sclerosis and am desperate for treatment. Can you help me? — *G.W., North Dakota*

A. A few patients with MS have been treated with intravenous H_2O_2 but not enough to come to any conclusions as to the efficacy of the treatment. I suggest that you contact IOMA (Send $5 and a written request for a list of doctors to P.O. Box 891954, Oklahoma City, OK 73189) and discuss your situation with a doctor familiar with this therapy. The treatment is quite safe.

I also suggest that you take "EWOT" — Exercise With Oxygen Therapy. This is accomplished by exercising on a stationary bicycle (or other exercise modality if the bike is too difficult), while breathing oxygen through a nasal cannula at six to eight liters a minute.

International Bio-Oxidative Medicine Foundation Doctor's List

Dear friend of oxidative medicine,

The International Bio-Oxidative Medicine Foundation is a small non-profit organization dedicated to preserve and advance oxidative medicine. I humbly and respectfully ask for any donation you can make to help this great organization bring oxidative therapies to the world. This way it can continue to serve you and others seeking such help. Please send your tax-deductible donations to IBOMF, P.O. Box 30006, Edmond, OK 73003. Your gifts are very much appreciated. If you have any questions regarding oxidative therapies or specific health issues, these should be directed to the physicians on this referral list

Yours for better health,

Robert Jay Rowen, MD
President, IOMA

ARIZONA

Jeff A. Baird, DO
1413 16th Street
Parker, AZ 85344
Ph: 928-669-9229
Fx: 928-669-8402

Garry F. Gordon, MD
Gordon Research Institute
708 E. Hwy 260, C-2, Suite F
Payson, AZ 85541
Ph: 928-472-4263
Fax: 928-474-3819
drgary@gordonresearch.com

Daniela Hutyrova, NMD
Pante Rhei Wellness & Rejuvenation
203 S. Candy Lane Suite 2B
Cottonwood, AZ 86326
Ph: 928-399-0636
Fax: 928-649-2024
drdanila@yahoo.com

Gordon Josephs, DO
CCUSA, LLC
7315 E. Evans Road
Scottsdale, AZ 85260
Ph: 480-998-9232
Fax: 480-998-1528
gjosephs@chelationcare.com

Charles D. Schwengel, DO
1215 E. Brown Road
Mesa, AZ 85203
Ph: 480-668-1448
Fax: 480-898-7323

Joseph Sherman, DO
54551 E. Herrara Drive
Phoenix, AZ 85054
Ph: 480-600-7621
Joedo3@juno.com

Sam Walters, DO
8070 E. Morgan Trail Suite 200
Scottsdale, AZ 85258
Ph: 480-946-9222
Fax: 946-946-9226

ARKANSAS

Melissa Taliaferro, MD
Leslie Medical Center
101 Cherry Street
Leslie, AR 72645
Ph: 870-447-2599

CALIFORNIA

Les Breitman, MD
Institute for Anti-Aging Med.
2023 W. Vista Way, Suite F
Vista, CA 92083
Ph: 760-439-9155
anti_aging22@hotmail.com

Joseph Chun, MD
201 S. Alvarado Street Suite 702
Los Angeles, CA 90057
Ph: 213-480-1475
Fax: 213-480-1416

Bryn Henderson, MD
954 West Foothill Blvd. Suite B
Upland, CA 91786
Ph: 909-985-8250

Bernard McGinity, MD
6945 Fair Oaks Blvd.
Carmichael, CA 95608
Ph: 916-485-4556
Fax: 916-485-1491

James Munson, MD
245 Terracina Blvd, Suite 209-C
Redlands, CA 92373
Ph: 909-793-2999

Philip J Reilly, MD
4800 Manzanita Ave., Suite 17
Carmichael, CA 95608
Ph: 916-488-9524
Fax: 916-488-9554

Robert Rowen, MD
2200 Country Club Drive Suite H
Santa Rosa, CA 95403
Ph: 707-571-7560
Fax: 707-571-8929

David A. Steenblock, DO
26381 Crown Valley Parkway, #130
Mission Viejo, CA 92961
Ph: 949-367-8870
Fax: 949-367-9779

David L. Stokesbury, MD
Advanced Magnetic
Research Institute
27652 Camino Capistrano Suite B
Laguna Niguel, CA 95403
Ph: 949-582-2057
Fax: 949-367-1716

Terri Su, MD
2200 Country Club Drive Suite H
Santa Rosa, CA 95403
Ph: 707-571-7560
Fax: 707-571-8929

John P. Toth, MD
2270 Bacon Street
Concord, CA 94520
Ph: 925-687-9447
Fax: 925-687-9483

COLORADO

Terry A. Grossman, MD
Frontier Medical Institute
2801 Youngfield Street #117
Golden, CO 80401
Ph: 303-233-4247
Fax: 303-233-4249

FLORIDA

Valerie G. Davis, MD
504 South Orange Street
New Smyrna Beach, FL 32168
Ph: 386-423-2218
Fax: 386-427-0980

Robert Erickson, MD
905 NW 56th Terrace, Suite B
Gainsville, FL 32605
Ph: 352-331-5138
Fax: 352-331-9399

Nelson Keaucek, MD
Life Family Practice
1501 US Hwy 441 N, #1702
The Villages, FL 32159
Ph: 352-750-4333
Fax: 352-750-2023

James E. Lemire, MD
6199 W. Gulf to Lake Hwy
Crystal River, FL 34429
Ph: 352-291-9459
jelemure@digitalusa.net

Gary L. Pynckel, DO
3840 Colonial Blvd
Fort Myers, FL 33912
Ph: 239-278-3377

Dean Silver, MD
9240 Bonita Beach Road, #2215
Bonita Springs, FL 34135
lifemd@earthlink.net

John Song, MD
Community Quick Medical
3660 20th Street
Vero Beach, FL 32960
Ph: 772-770-2070
Fax: 772-567-4597

Daniel Tucker, MD
1411 N. Flagler Drive, # 6700
West Palm Beach, FL 33401
Ph: 561-835-0055
Fax: 561-835-1742

GEORGIA

Robert A. Burkich, MD
148 Scruggs Road
Ringgold, GA 30736
Ph: 706-891-1200
Fax: 706-891-1202

Ralph G. Ellis, Jr., MD
Coastal Georgia Health
Research Institute
158 Scranton Connector Blvd.
Brunswick, GA 31525
Ph: 912-280-0304

ILLINOIS

Terrence J. Bugno, MD
East West Integrative Medicine
1201 Main Street, Rte., 31
Algonquin, IL 60102
Ph: 847-756-4540

Ross A. Hauser, MD
Caring Medical
715 Lake Street, Suite #600
Oak Park, IL 60301
Ph: 708-848-7789
Fax: 708-848-7763
drhauser@caringmedical.com

Thomas L. Hesselink, MD
888 S. Edgelawn Drive
Aurora, IL 60506
Ph: 630-844-0011
Fax: 630-844-0500
hesselink@pol.net

INDIANA

Marvin Dziabis, MD
Health Restoration Clinic
107 West Seventh Street
North Manchester, IN 46962
Ph: 260-982-1400
Fax: 260-982-1700
mdziabis@cltnet.com

Janice M. Smith, MD
215 East Mishawaka
Mishawaka, IN 46545
Ph: 574-258-1111
Fax: 574-255-5156

William D. Stimack, NMD
Nature's Gifts
4004 Campbell Street
Valparaiso, IN 46385
Ph: 219-531-0241
Fax: 219-465-5998

Arthur Sumrall, MD
Longevity Institute Of Indiana
9292 N. Meridian Street
Indianapolis, IN 46260
Ph: 317-574-1677
Fax: 317-574-1688

Charles Turner, MD
3554 Promenade Parkway,
Suite H
Lafayette, IN 47909
Ph: 765-471-1100
Fax: 765-471-1009

KANSAS

George Watson, DO
Park City Medical Center
425 East 61st N, Suite 2
Park City, KS 67219
Ph: 316-744-3400
Fax: 316-744-3800

MASSACHUSETTS

Carol Englender, MD
160 Speen Street, #203
Framingham, MA 01701
Ph: 508-875-0875

Nutrition Consultant's
of Cape Cod
P.O. Box 933
South Yarmouth, MA 02664
Ph: 508-760-2423
preventivemedicine@onemain.com

MICHIGAN

Vahagn Agobabian, DO
28 North Saginaw, Suite 1105
Pontiac, MI 48342
Ph: 248-334-2424
Fax: 248-334-2924
agbabian@hotmail.com

Tammy Born, DO
Born Preventive Health Care
3700 52nd Street, S.E.
Grand Rapids, MI 49512
Ph: 616-656-3700
Fax: 616-656-3701
tborn@bornclinic.com

David Nibbling, DO
3918 W. Saint
Lansing, MI
Ph: 517-323-1833
Fax: 517-323-1842

MISSOURI

Harry Osaghaemorgan, MD
Preventive/Anti-Aging Med.
8420 Delmar Boulevard
University City, MO 63124
Ph: 314-993-3002
Fax: 314-993-3013

NEBRASKA

J. William LaValley, MD
Medical Wellness Center
P.O. Box 2020
Chester, NS B0J 1J0
Ph: 902-275-4555
Fax: 902-275-4555

NEVADA

Carol Barlow, MD, HMD
Allergy Institute of Nevada
3280 N. Rainbow Blvd.
Las Vegas, NV 89108
Ph: 702-731-3117
Fax: 702-731-3840

David A. Edwards, MD, HMD
Bio Health Center
615 Sierra Rose Drive
Reno, NV 89511
Ph: 775-828-4055
Fax: 775-808-4255
info@biohealthcenter.com

Robbie Grant, DO
395 W. Minor Street
Winnemucca, NV 89445
Ph: 775-623-6622
Fax: 775-623-0979
rigrant@fiberpipe.net

Robert D. Milne, MD
Milne Medical Center
2110 Pinto Lane
Las Vegas, NV 89106
Ph: 702-385-1393
Fax: 702-385-4170
mmc@lvcm.com

NEW JERSEY

Ivan Krohn, MD
1140 Burnt Tavern Road
Brick, NJ 08724
Ph: 732-785-2670
Fax: 732-785-2673

NEW MEXICO

Ralph J. Luciani, DO
Albuquerque Clinic
10601 Lomas Blvd. NE, Suite 103
Albuquerque, NM 87112
Ph: 505-298-5995
Fax: 505-298-2940

NEW YORK

Mitchell Kurk, MD
Lawrence Family Medical
310 Broadway
Lawrence, NY 11559
drkurk@hotmail.com

NORTH CAROLINA

Dennis Fera, MD
Holistic Health & Medicine
1000 Corporate Drive, #209
Hillsborough, NC 27278
Ph: 919-732-2287
Fax: 919-732-3176
holistic-med@mindspring.com

John C. Pittman, MD
The Carolina Center
4505 Fair Meadow Lane, #111
Raleigh, NC 27607
Ph: 919-571-4391
Fax: 919-571-8968
info@carolinacenter.com

OHIO

Theodore J. Cole, DO
Cole Center for Healing
11974 Lebanon Road, Suite 228
Sharonville, OH 45241
Ph: 513-563-4321
tedcole@medscape.com

OKLAHOMA

Douglas B. Cook, DC
OK Health & Wellness Center
1108 N. Washington
Weatherford, OK 73096
Ph: 580-774-2214
Fax: 580-774-2843

Genesis Medical Research
Foundation
5419 South Western
Oklahoma City, OK 73109
Ph: 405-634-7855
Fax: 405-634-0778

Michael Taylor, DC
Marion Medical
3808-B East 51st Street
Tulsa, OK 74135
Ph: 918-749-3797
Fax: 918-749-1536
dr.taylor@healinginc.net

OREGON

Franklin H. Ross, Jr., MD
Integrated Health Care
565 A Street
Ashland, OR 97520
Ph: 541-482-7007
Fax: 541-482-5123

Terence H. Young, MD
Cornerstone Clinic
1205 Wallace Road, NW
Salem, OR 97304
Ph: 503-371-1558
Fax: 503-375-3866

PENNSYLVANIA

Andrew Lipton, DO
Narberth Family Medicine
822 Montgomery Avenue, #315
Narberth, PA 19072
Ph: 610-667-4601
Fax: 610-667-6414

SOUTH CAROLINA

Rodrigo Rojas, MD
1314 Fording Island Road
Bluffton, SC 29910
Ph: 843-757-8717

TENNESSEE

Joseph Rich, MD
Center for Environment & Int. Med.
9217 Parkwest Blvd., Suite E-1
Knoxville, TN 37923
Ph: 865-694-9553
Fax: 865-594-7658
mascots@pol.net

TEXAS

Frank J. Morales, MD, NMD
Rio Valley Medical Center
1474 West Price Road, #450
Brownsville, TX 78520
Ph: 956-592-5584
drfrank59@gmail.com

Rosa Maria Morales, DDS, NMD
Rio Valley Medical Center
1474 West Price Road, #450
Brownsville, TX 78520
Ph: 956-592-5585

Vladimir Rizov, MD
Austin Rejuvenation Center
911 West Anderson Lane,
Suite 205
Austin, TX 78757
info@newvitality.com

Texas Institute of
Functional Medicine
4001 McEwen Road, Suite 102
Dallas, TX 75244
Ph: 972-239-6317
Fax: 972-490-7438

Michael Truman, DO
Holistic Wellness Center
2401 Canton Drive
Fort Worth, TX 76112
Ph: 817-446-5500
Fax: 817-446-5509
mtruman981@aol.com

VIRGINIA

E. Aubrey Murden, MD
Alternative Integrated Med.
4020 Raintree Road, Suite C
Chesapeake, VA 23321
Ph: 757-488-9900
Fax: 757-405-3025
tidewater-ent@edifax.com

WASHINGTON

Thomas Dorman, MD
2505 South 320th Street, #100
Federal Way, WA 98003
Ph: 253-529-3050

Donald Lee McCabe, DO
Freeland Medical Center
1689 East Main Street
Freeland, WA 98249
Ph: 360-331-4424
Fax: 360-331-1679
mccabe@whedbev.com

Jon Mundall, MD
111 North Columbia Avenue
Connell, WA 99326
Ph: 509-234-7766
Fax: 509-234-4320

WISCONSIN

Steven G. Meress, DO
Fox Valley Wellness Center
180 Knights Way
Fond du Lac, WI 54935
Ph: 920-922-5433
Fax: 920-922-5422

Carol Uebelacker, MD
700 Milwaukee Street
Delafield, WI 53018
Ph: 262-646-4600
Fax: 262-646-4215

INTERNATIONAL

CANANDA

Eric Arrata, ND
Integrative Medicine Institute
170, 1402 Alberta T2N-1B9
Ph: 403-233-0917
Fax: 403-233-0911

Robert J. Ewing, ND
Clearbrook Clinic
2431 Clearbrook Road
Abbotsford, BC V2T 2X9
Ph: 604-504-1978
Fax: 604-504-1868
robertewing@shaw.ca

Donn Gaudin, PhD, MD
C.C.I.H.S.
30 Sword Street
Toronto, Ont. M5A 3N2

Richard Russell Johnson, MD
Johnson's Holistix, #222
4935 40th Avenue, NW
Calgary, AB T3A 2N1
Ph: 403-202-0724
Fax: 403-247-0711
holstix@telusplanet.net

Tarit Kanungo, MBBS
180 Vine Street
St. Catharine's, Ontario,
Suite 105B
Ph: 905-682-7555
Fax: 905-682-7446

J. William LaValley, MD
Medical Wellness Centre
P.O. Box 2020
Chester, NS B0J 1J0
Ph: 902-275-4555
Fax: 902-275-4555

Garrett G. Swetlekoff, ND
160-1855 Kirschner Road
Kelowna, BC V1Y 4N7
Ph: 250-868-2205

GERMANY

John G. Ionescu, PhD
Spezialklinik Neukirchen
Krankenhausstr. 9
Neukirchen b.Hl.Blut 93454
GERMANY
Ph: 011-49-9947-28122
Fx: 011-49-9947-28109
info@allergieklinik.de

IRELAND

Dr. Mary Dunphy
Cork Road Clinic
Carrigaline, CO Cork
Ph: 011-021-4971177
Fax: 011-021-4371417
drdunphy@eircour.net

JAPAN

Hideo Suzuki, MD
1233 Haniya Sanbu Machi
Sanbugun, Chiba 2891223
suuhideo@hotmail.com

Tadashi Mitsuo, MD
8-6-9 Akasaka
#801 Partyru Akasaka
Minato-ku Tokio, 107-0052

MEXICO

Frank J. Morales, MD
Avenida Coahulila #300
Progreso, Tamaulipas Mexico
Ph: 011-52-89-99-37-01-59

Rosa Maria Morales, DDS
Avenida Coahulila #300
Progreso, Tamaulipas Mexico
Ph: 011-52-89-99-37-01-59

Appendix II

Therapeutic Uses of H$_2$O$_2$

Intravenous hydrogen peroxide is a *universal treatment* because it increases oxygen available to the tissues; it has a truly remarkable range of effectiveness. Because the treatment increases oxygen availablitity, whether due to the direct effect of the oxygen produced by the hydrogen peroxide or the secondary manufacturing of oxygen by the body in response to the hydrogen peroxide, it is a basic treatment that can be used with almost any other therapy in almost any disease. The peroxide is always given separately and not mixed with other agents.

Although much more clinical work needs to be done, the following disease conditions and infecting agents are candidates for hydrogen peroxide therapy:

Peripheral Vascular Disease

Cerebral Vascular Disease

Alzheimer's

Cardiovascular Disease

Coronary Spasm (angina)

Cardioconversion

Arrhythmias

Chronic Obstructive Pulmonary Disease

Emphysema

Asthma

Influenza

Herpes Zoster

Herpes Simplex

Temporal Arteritis

Systemic Chronic Candidiasis

Chronic Recurrent Ebstein-Barr Infection

Diabetes Type II
HIV infections
Metastatic Carcinoma
Multiple Sclerosis
Rheumatoid Arthritis
Acute and Chronic viral infections
Chronic unresponsive bacterial infection
Parasitic infections
Parkinsonism
Migraine headaches
Cluster headaches
Vascular headaches
Chronic pain syndromes (multiple etiologies)
Environmental allergy reactions (Universal)

BACTERIA (Numbers refer to bibliography)
Legionella pneumophila (62)
Treponema pallidum (63)
Escherichia coli (64)
Salmonella typhimurium (65)
Mycobacterium leprae (66)
Staphylococcus aureus (67)
Pseudomonas aeruginosa (68)
Campylobacter jejuni (69)
Salmonella typhi (70)
Group B Streptococci (71)
Bacillus cereus (72)
Actinobacillus actinomycetermoncomitans (73)
Bacteroides (74)
Neisseria gonorrhoeae (75)

FUNGI
Histoplasma capsulatum (76)
Candida albicans (77)

Coccidioides (78)
Paraoccidioides (78)
Blastomyces (78)
Sporothrix (78)
Mucoraceae (78)
Aspergillus fumigatus (79)
Coccidioides immitis (80)

PARASITES

Pneumocystis carinii (81)
Plasmodium yoelii (82)
Plasmodium berghei (82)
Toxoplasma gondii (83)
Nippostrongycus brasiliensis (84)
Naegleria fowleri (85)
Leishmania major (86)
Schistosoma mansoni (87)
Chlamydia psittaci (88)
Trichomonas vaginalis (89)
Tepanosoma cruzi (90)
Endameba histolytica (91)

TUMOR TYPES

Enrlich carinoma (94)
Neuroblastoma (95)

VIRUSES

Human Immunodeficiency Virus (92)
Cytomegalovirus (67)
Lymphocytic choriomeningitis virus (93)
Tacaribe virus (93)

Many studies within the body and the laboratory have shown that peroxide will kill bacteria, fungi, parasites, viruses and has been shown to destroy certain tumors. As mentioned, much more work needs to be done, but peroxide is certainly a universal agent which can almost always be tried for an illness, often with great success.

As Dr. Farr has so apply put it: "No distinct group of patients or classifications of disease at this time can be considered the 'proper selections.' Since intravenous infusions of hydrogen peroxide provide oxygenation to highly toxic tissue, kill or inhibit certain bacteria, yeast, viruses, protozoa and parasites, and, since it has a stimulatory effect on the immune system, many different pathological conditions seem to respond to intravenous peroxide therapy."

Appendix III

Metabolic and Physiological Effects of Peroxide Healing

Numerous physiological effects are attributed to hydrogen peroxide and documented in the literature. Some of these effects may be broadly categorized as follows:

1. Pulmonary

   a. Increased oxygenation (37) — Increased oxygenation up to 12 atmospheres have been reported in tissue following both the intra-venous and intra-arterial infusions of H_2O_2.

   b. Alveolar debridement (31) — Alveolar debridement occurs due to the action of oxygen, generated by intravenous hydrogen peroxide, as it diffuses from the pulmonary veins into the alveolar space. The retrograde diffusing oxygen undermines mucous or other accumulated materials in the alveolus, promoting expectoration.

2. Metabolic Rate

   a. Hormonal effect

   Several hormonal effects have been reported to be regulated by the action of H_2O_2. Examples are:

   1. Iodination of thyroglobin (13)
   2. Production of thyronine (13)
   3. Progesterone production (107)
   4. Inhibition of bioamines (108); dopamine, noradrenalin and serotonin
   5. Prostaglandin synthesis (46, 47, 109)
   6. Dopamine metabolism (110)

    7. Regulates Reticulum Calcium Transport (111)

  b. Stimulation of Oxidative Enzyme System Hydrogen Peroxide directly and indirectly stimulates oxidative enzyme systems. Micromolar amounts of infused H_2O_2 have been found to increase oxidative enzymatic activity to the maximum rate of reaction. This enzymatic stimulation influences many different metabolic pathways.

    1. Increases GSH oxidation to GSSG, which increases ATP production (112)

    2. Activities Hexose Monophosphate Shunt (41)

    3. Alters Na-KATPase activity (12)

    4. Regulates cellular (113) and mitochrondial (15) membrane transport

    5. Regulates thermogenic control (11)

3. Vascular Response

  a. Vasodilation

    1. Dilation of peripheral vessels (31)

    2. Dilation of coronary vessels (114)

    3. Aortic strip relaxation response (115)

    4. Cerebral arteriolar dilation (116, 117)

    5. Pulmonary arterial relaxation (118)

  b. Vasoconstriction — Essential Hypertension effect (31) — Patients with severe essential hypertension have been reported to have a vasoconstriction response to infusions instead of vasodilation, which usually occurs.

4. Glucose Utilization

  a. H_2O_2 mimics insulin (16)

  b. Increases glycogen production from glucose (119)

  c. Type II Diabetes Mellitus stabilized with H_2O_2 infusions (120)

5. Granulocyte Response

    a. Depressed granulocytes after treatment, then rebound measured after 24 hours (31)

    b. Secondary resistance to peroxide after exposure (109)

    c. Alterations of T-4/T-8 ratio with increase of T-4 Helper cells (28)

6. Immune Response

    a. Stimulates Monocytes (92)

    b. Stimulates T-Helper cells (109)

    c. Stimulates Gamma Interferon production (58)

    d. Decreases B-cell activity (121)

    e. Responsible for immunoregulation (58)

    f. Regulates inflammatory response (122)

Notes

Foreword
1. Nathan and Cohn, *Journal of Experimental Medicine*, 1981;154:1539-1553.

Introduction
1. *Orange County Register*, November 12, 1982.

2. Journal of the American Medical Association, April 11, 1914.

3. Donsbach, *Health Freedom News*, pp. 24, August 1987.

Chapter 1
1. Singh, et,al, *The Lancet, May* 18, 1940; pp. 922.

2. *Lancet*, August 19, 1916.

3. *Demarquay: Essaide Pneumatologic Medicale*, Paris, 1886, p. 637.

4. *British Medical Journal*, December 14, 1985 pp. 1706.

Chapter 2
1. MacNaughton, *International Journal of Radiation Biology*, 1971; 19: 405-413.

2. Rowley and Halliwell, *Clinical Science*, 1983; 64:649-653.

3. Ackerman and Brinkley, *Surgery,* 1968.

4. Farr, *Journal of the American College for the Advancement of Medicine*, 1987.

5. Farr, *Protocol for the Intravenous Administration of Hydrogen Peroxide*, 1987.

6. Finney, et al, *Angiology,* 1966; 17:223-228.

7. J. Hug (London), August, 1986, 97(1), pp. 61.

8. *Can. J. Microbiol.*, December 1984, 30(12), pp. 1467.

9. Ibid.

10. Govoni, et al, *Arn. J. Roent.*, 71:235-238, 1954.

Chapter 3

1. *J. Clin. Period.*, 1979, 6:15.

2. Docknell, *Inf. / Immunol.*, January 1983, pp. 456.

3. Urschel, *Dis. of Chest,* 1967;51:180-192.

4. Finney, et al, *Ann. N.Y. Acad. of Science,* 1967;151:231-241.

5. Urschel, *Circulation,* 1965, 31 (supplement II):203-210.

6. Mallams, Finney & Balla, *Southern Medical Journal,* March 1962.

Chapter 4

1. Jay, et al, *Tex. Rep. Biol. & Med.*, 22:102,1964.

2. Finney, et al, *Angiology,* 16:62, 1965.

3. Gray, *Radiation Biology,* Ch. 10, pp. 76, Butterworth Press, London 1959, Howard, Nature (London), 207, 776, 1965.

4. Meyer, et al, *J. Clin. Gastro.,* 3:31-35, 1981.

5. *J. Inorgan Biochem,* 1989 Jan., 35(1):55-69.

6. *IBOM Newsletter, Vol.* I, #1.

Chapter 5

1. Farber, et al, *Journal of Immunology,* 1984;132. (5):2543 1984;132.

2. Farr, *Proceedings of the First International Conference on Bio-Oxidative Medicine,* 1989: in publication.

Chapter 6

1. Lorencz, et. al., 31st Ann. Meeting, Fed. Am. Soc Exp. Bio., May 20, 1947.

Chapter 7

1. Brummelkamp, *N.Y. Academy of Science,* 177, 688.

2. *J. Cancer Res. Clin. Oncol.*, 1986,11(2), pp. 93.

3. *J. Gen. Microbiol.,* October 1976, 96(2), pp. *401.*

4. *In-Vitro,* August 1978,14(8), pp. 715.

5. *Br. J. Hematol.*, January 1979, 41(1), pp. *49.*

6. *"Appl., Environ.", Microbiol.,* August 1980, *40(2), pp.* 337.

7. Ibid.

8. *Biotechnol. Bioeng.,* March 1977, 19(3), pp. 413.

9. *Infection & Immunity,* June 1985, pp. 607-10.

10. *N.Y. Acad. Sci.,* date unknown.

11. Siderova, et al, Toksikol 7, #3, pp. 39, 1944.

12. *Consumer Reports,* February 1992.

13. See Monograph on Lithia Springs water. Order from: Lithia Springs Water Co., 2910 Bankhead Highway, Lithia Springs, GA 30057. Send $2.00 for postage and handling (for two copies).

14. *Western Journal of Medicine,* February 1990, 152 *Surgery,* 1988; 103: 389-397

Chapter 8

1. William Campbell Douglass, M.D., *Into the Light,* Second Opinion Publishing, P.O. Box 467939, Atlanta, Georgia 31146-7939, 800-728-2288 or 404-399-5617.

Chapter 9

1. *Coastweek,* July 28, 1989.

2. *World Health Magazine,* March 1989.

Bibliography

For doctors and scientists interested in verifying the material in this book we recommend the following references:

1. Oliver TH, Cantab BC, and Murphy DV: Influenzal Pneumonia: The Intravenous Injection of Hydrogen Peroxide. *Lancet* 1920; 1: 432-433.

2. Tsai SK, Lee TY, Mok MS: Gas Embolism Produced by Hydrogen Peroxide Irrigation of an Anal Fistula During Anesthesia. *Anesthesiology* 1985; 63: 316-317.

3. Shah J, Pedemonte MS, Wilcock MM: Hydrogen Peroxide May Cause Venous Oxygen Embolism. *Anesthesiology* 1984; 61:631-632.

4. Sleigh J, Linter SPK: Hazards of Hydrogen Peroxide. *British Med J* 1985; 291:1706.

5. Meyer CT, Brand M, DeLuca VA, et al: Hydrogen Peroxide Colitis: A Report of Three Patients. *J Clin Gastroenterol* 1981;3:31-35.

6. Shenep JL, Stokes DC, Hughes WT: Lack of Antibacterial Activity After Intravenous Hydrogen Peroxide Infusion in Experimental Escherichia coli Sepses. *Infect. Immun.* 1985; 48:607-610.

7. Dockrell HM and Playfair JH: Killing of Blood-Stage Murine Malaria Parasites by Hydrogen Peroxide. *Infect. Immun.* 1983;39:456-459.

8. Weiss SJ, Young J, LoBuglio A, et al: Role of Hydrogen Peroxide in Neutrophil-Mediated Destruction of Cultured Endothelial Cells. *J. Clin. Invest.* 1981; 68: 714-721.

9. Root RK, Metcalf J, Oshino N, et al: H_2O_2 Release from Human Granulocytes during Phagocytosis. *J. Clin. Invest.* 1975;55:945-955.

10. Root RK and Metcalf JA: H_2O_2 Release from Human Granulocytes during Phagocytosis. *J. Clin. Invest.* 1977;60: 1266-1279.

11. Ramasarma T: Generation of H_2O_2 in Biomembranes. *Biochemica et Biophysica ACTA* 1982; 694: 69-93.

12. Garner MH, Garner WH, Spector A: Kinetic Cooperativity Change after H_2O_2 Modification of (Na,K)-ATPase, *J. Biolog. Chem.* 1984; 259: 7712-7718.

13. Wildberger E, Kohler H, Jenzer H, et al: Inactivation of Peroxidase and Glucose Oxidase by H_2O_2 and Iodide during In Vitro Thyroglobulin Iodination. *Mol Cell Endocrinol* 1986; 46(2): 149-154.

14. Swaroop A and Ramasarma T: Heat Exposure and Hypothyroid Conditions Decrease Hydrogen Peroxide Production Generation in Liver Mitochrondia. *J. Biochem.* 1985; 226(2): 403-8.

15. Nelson DH and Murray DK: Dexamethasone Inhibition of Hydrogen Peroxide-stimulated Glucose Transport. *Endocrinology* 1987; 120(1): 156-159.

16. Helm AU and Gunn J: The Effect of Insulinomimetic Agents on Protein Degradation in H-35 Hepatoma Cells. *Mol. Cell. Biochem.* 1986; 71(2): 159-166.

17. Jay BE, Finney JW, Balla GA, et al: The Supersaturation of Biologic Fluids with Oxygen by the Decomposition of Hydrogen Peroxide. *Texas Rpts. Biol and Med* 1964; 22: 106-109.

18. Balla GA, Finney JW, Aronoff BL, et al: Use of Intraarterial Hydrogen Peroxide to Promote Wound Healing. An~ J. Surg. 1964;108:621-629.

19. Fuson RL, Kylstra JA, Hochstein P, et al: Intravenous Hydrogen Peroxide Infusion as a Means of Extrapulmonary Oxygenation. *Clin. Res.* 1967;15: 74.

20. Finney JW, Balla GA, Race GJ, et al: Peripheral Blood Changes in Humans and Experimental Animals Following the Infusion of Hydrogen Peroxide into the Carotid Artery. *Angio* 1965; 16:62-66.

21. Mallams JT, Finney JW, and Balla GA: The Use of Hydrogen Peroxide As A Source of Oxygen in A Regional Intra-Arterial Infusion System. *So. M. J.* 1962; 55: 230-232.

22. Lorincz AL, Jacoby JJ, Livingstone MM: Studies on the Parenteral Administration of Hydrogen Peroxide. Anesthesiology 1948; 9: 162-174. .

23. Rowley DA and Halliwell B: Formation of Hydroxyl Radicals from Hydrogen Peroxide and Iron Salts by Superoxide and Ascorbate-dependent Mechanisms: Relevance to the Pathology of Rheumatoid Disease. *Clin. Sci.* 1983; 64: 649-653.

24. MacNaughton JI: Regional Oxygenation and Radiotherapy: A Study of the Degradation of Infused Hydrogen Peroxide. II. Measurement of Decomposition of H_2O_2 Infused Into Flowing Blood. *Int. J. Radiat. Biol.* 1971;19: 415-426.

25. MacNaughton JI: Regional Oxygenation and Radiotherapy: A Study of the Degradation of Infused Hydrogen Peroxide. I. Infusate Mixing. *Int. J. Radiat. Biol.* 1971;19: 405-413.

26. Snyder LM, Fortier NL, Trainor J, et al: Effect of Hydrogen Peroxide Exposure on Normal Human Erythrocyte Deformability, Morphology, Surfact Characteristics, and Spectrin-Hemoglobin Cross-Linking. *J. Clin. Invest.* 1985; 76: 1971-1977.

27. Minotti G and Aust SD: The Requirement for Iron (III) in the Initiation of Lipid Peroxidation by Iron(II) and Hydrogen Peroxide. J. Biol. Chem. 1987: 262(3): 1098-104.

28. Farr CH: Possible Therapeutic Value of Intravenous Hydrogen Peroxide. Second International Symposium; Chelating Agents in Pharmacology, Toxicology and Therapeutics 1987; Charles University, Pilsen, Czechoslovak (In press).

29. Diez-Marques ML, Lucio-Cazana FJ and Rodriquez Puyol M: In-vitro Response of Erythrocytes to Alphatocopherol Exposure. Int. J. Vita~, Nutr., Res

1986; 56(3): 311-315.

30. Johnson RJR, Froese G, Khodadad M, et al: Hydrogen Peroxide and radiotherapy. Bubble Formation in Blood. *Br. J. Radiol.* 1968; 41: 749-754.

31. Farr CH: The Therapeutic Use of Intravenous Hydrogen Peroxide (Monograph). Genesis Medical Center, Oklahoma City, OK 73120, Jan. 1987.

32. Finney JW, Jay BE, Race GJ, et al: Removal of Cholesterol and Other Lipids from Experimental Animal and Human Atheromatous Arteries by Dilute Hydrogen Peroxide. *Angiology* 1966; 17: 223-228.

33. Urschel HE Jr: Cardiovascular Effects of Hydrogen Peroxide: Current Status. *Dis. of Chest* 1967; 51:180-192.

34. Finney JW, Balla GA, Race GJ, et al: Peripheral Blood Changes in Humans and Experimental Animals Following the Infusion of Hydrogen Peroxide into the Carotid Artery. *Angio.* 1965; 16: 62-66.

35. Finney JW, Urschel HC, Balla GA, et al: Protection of the Ischemic Heart with DMSO Alone or DMSO with Hydrogen Peroxide. *Ann. NY Acad. Sci.* 1967;151: 231-241.

36. Urschel HC, Finney JW, Morale AR, et al: Cardiac Resuscitation with Hydrogen Peroxide. *Circ.* 1965; 31 (suppl II); II-210.

37. Ackerman NB, Brinkley FB: Comparison of Effects on Tissue Oxygenation of Hyperbaric Oxygen and Intravascular Hydrogen Peroxide. *Sur.* 1968; 63: 285-290.

38. Germon PA, Faust DS, Brady, LW: Comparison of Arterial and Tissue Oxygen Measurements in Humans Receiving Regional Hydrogen Peroxide Infusions and Oxygen Inhalation. *Radiology* 1968; 91: 669-672.

39. Germon PA, Faust DS, Rosenthal A, et al: Regional Arterial and Tissue Oxygen Tensions in Man During Regional Infusion with Hydrogen Peroxide Solutions. *Radiology* 1967; 88:589-591.

40. Farr CH: Physiological and Biochemical Responses to Intravenous Hydrogen Peroxide in Man. *J. ACAM* 1987; (In Press).

41. Hothersall JD, Greenbaum AL, McLean P: The Functional Significance of the Pentose Phosphate Pathway in Synaptosomes: Protection Against Peroxidative Damage by Catecholamines and Oxidants. *J. Neurochem.* 1982; 39:13252.

42. Cranne D, Haussinger D, Sies H: Rise of Coenzyme A-Glutathione Mixed Disulfide during Hydroperoxide Metabolism in Perfused Rat Liver. *Euo. J. Biochem.* 1982; 127: 575-578.

43. Wrigglesworth JM: Formation and Reduction of a 'Peroxy' Intermediate of Cytochrome C Oxidase by Hydrogen Peroxide. *Biochem. J.* 1984; 217; 715-719.

44. Gorren AC, Dekker H and Wever R: Kinetic Investigations of the Reactions of Cytochrome C Oxidase with Hydrogen Peroxide. *Biochem. Biophys. Acta.* 1986; 852(1): 81-92.

45. Del Maestro RF, Thaw HH, Bjork J, et al: Free Radicals as Mediators of Tissue Injury. *Acta Physiol. Scand.* 1980; 492(supple):43-57.

46. Yamaja Setty BN, Jurek E, Ganley C, et al: Effects of Hydrogen Peroxide on Vascular Arachidonic Acid Metabolism. *Prostag. Leuko. Med* 1984;14: 205-213.

47. Polgar P, Taylor L: Stimulation of Prostaglandin Synthesis by Ascorbic Acid via EIydrogen Peroxide Formation. *Prostag* 1980;19:693.

48. Marshall PJ and Lands WE: In Vitro Formation of Activators for Prostaglandin Synthesis by Neutrophils and Macrophages from Humans and Guinea Pigs. *J. Lab. Clin. Med.* 1986;108(6):525-534.

49. Tappel AL: Lipid Peroxidation Damage to Cell Component. *Fed Proc.* 1973; 32:1870.

50. Shimada O and Yashuda H: Lipid Peroxidation and its Inhibition by Tinoridine. *Biochem. Biophys. ACTA* 1979; 572: 531.

51. Morehouse LA, Tien M, Bucher JR, et al: Effect of Hydrogen Peroxide on the Initiation of Microsomal Lipid Peroxidation. *Biochem. Pharm.* 1983; 32:123-127.

52. Harrison JF and Schultz J: Studies on the Chlorinating Activity of Myeloperoxidase. *J. Biol. Chem.* 1976; 251:13711374.

53. Zgliczynski JM, Selvaraj RJ, Paul BB, et al: Chlorination by the Myeloperoxidase-H_2O_2-C1 antimicrobial system at Acid and Neutral pH. *Proc. Soc. Exp. Biol. Med* .1977;154: 418-422.

54. Kiebanoff SJ: Oxygen Metabolism and the Toxic Properties of Phagocytes. *Ann. Intern. Med.* 1980; 93: 480-489.

55. Slivka A, LoBuglio AF, Weiss SJ: A Potential Role for Hypochlorous Acid in Granulocyte-Mediated Tumor Cell Cytotoxicity. *Blood* 1980; 55: 347-350.

56. Thomas EL: Myeloperoxidase, Hydrogen Peroxide, Chloride Antimicrobial System: Nitrogen-Chlorine Derivatives of Bacterial Components in Bacterial Action against Eschericia coli. *Infec. Immun.* 1979; 23: 522-531.

57. Nathan CF and Cohn ZA: Antitumor Effects of Hydrogen Peroxide in Vivo. *J. Exp. Med.* 1981; 154:1539-1553.

58. Munakata T, Semba U, Shibuya Y, et al: Induction of Interferon-gamma Production by Human Natural Killer Cells Stimulated by Hydrogen Peroxide. *J. Immunol.* 1985;134(4): 2449-2455.

59. Lebedev LV, Levin AO, Romankova MP, et al: Regional Oxygenation in the Treatment of Severe Destructive Forms of Obliterating Diseases of the Extremity Arteries. *Vestn Khir* 1984;132:85-88.

60. Gusak VK, Klioner LI, Belinski VE, et al: Possibilities of Using Weak Solutions of Hydrogen Peroxide in the Treatment of Experimental Ischemia of the Lower Extremities. *Klin Khir* 1986;7:31-33.

61. Urschel HC, Finney JW, Dyll LM, et al: Treatment of Artheriosclerotic Obstructive Cerebrovascular Disease with Hydrogen Peroxide. *Vas. Serg.* 1967;1: 77-81.

62. Jepras RI and Fitzgeorge RB: The Effect of Oxygen-dependent Antimicrobial Systems on Strains of Legionella Pneumophila of Different Virulence. *J. Hyg.* (Lond) 1986; 97(1):61-9.

63. Steiner BM, Wong GH, Sutrave P, et al: Oxygen Toxicity in Treponema Pallidum: Deoxyribonucleic Acid Singlestranded Breakage Induced by Low Doses of Hydrogen Peroxide. *Can. J. Microbiol.* 1984; 30(12): 1467-76.

64. Brandi G, Sestili P, Pedrini MA, et al: The Effect of Temperature or Anoxia on Escherichia Coli Killing Induced by Hydrogen Peroxide. *Mutat Res.* 1987; 190(4): 237-40.

65. Norkus EP, Kuenzig W, Conney AH: Studies on the Mutagenic Activity of Ascorbic Acid in Vitro and in Vivo. *Mutat. Res.* 1983;117(1): 183-9.

66. Klebanoff SJ and Shepard CC: Toxic Effect of the Peroxidase-hydrogen peroxide-halide Antimicrobial System on Mycobacterium leprae. *Infect. Immun.* 1984; 44(2): 534-6.

67. Miller SA, Bia FJ, Coleman DL, et al: Pulmonary Macrophage Function During Experimental Cytomegalovirus Interstitial Pneumonia. *Infect. Immun.* 1985; 47(1): 211-6.

68. Belotskii SM, Filiudova OB, Pashutin SB, et al: Chemiluminescence of Human Neutrophils as Affected by Opportunistic Microbes. *Zh. Mikrobiol. Epidemiol. Immunobiol.* 1986; Mar (3): 89-92.

69. Moran AP and Upton ME: Effect of Medium Supplements, Illumination and Superoxide Dismutase on the Production of Coccoid Forms of Campylobacter jejuni ATCC29428. *J. Appl. Bacteriol.* 1987; 62(1): 43-51.

70. Looney RJ and Steigbigel RT: Role of the Vi Antigen

of Salmonella typhi in Resistance to Host Defense In Vitro. *J. Lab. Clin. Med.* 1986;108(5): 506-16.

71. Wilson CB and Weaver WM: Comparative Susceptibility of Group B Streptococci and Staphylococcus aureus to Killing by Oxygen Metabolites. *J. Infect. Dis.* 1985;152(2): 323-9.

72. Tenovuo J, Makinen K, Sievers G: Antibacterial Effect of Lactoperoxidase and Myeloperoxidase Against Bacillus cereus. *Antimicrob. Agents Chemother.* 1985; 27(1): 96-101.

73. Miyasaki KT, Wilson ME, Genco RJ: Killing of Actinobacillus actinomycetemcomitans by the Human Neutrophil Myeloperoxidase-hydrogen peroxide-chloride System. *Infect. Immun.* 1986; 53(1): 161-5.

74. Rotstein OD, Nasmith PE, Grinstein S: The Bacteroides Byproduct Succinic Acid Inhibits Neutrophil Respiratory Burst by Reducing Intracellular pH. *Infect. Immun.* 1987; 55(4): 864-70.

75. Archibald FS and Duong MN: Superoxide Dismutase and Oxygen Toxicity Defenses in the Genus Neisseria. *Infect. Immun.* 1986; 51(2): 631-41.

76. Howard DH: Studies on the Catalase of Histoplasma Capsulatum. *Infect. Immun.* 1983; 39(3):1161-6.

77. Sasada M, Kubo A, Nishimura T, et al: Candidacidal Activity of Monocyte-derived Human Macrophages: Relationship between Candida Killing and Oxygen Radical Generation by Human Macrophages. *J. Leukocyte Biol.* 1987; 41(4): 289-94.

78. Schaffner A, Davis CE, Schaffner T, et al: In Vitro Susceptibility of Fungi to Killing by Neutrophil Granulocytes Discriminates Between Primary Pathogenicity and Opportunism. *J. Clin. Invest.* 1986; 78(2): 511-24.

79. Levitz SM and Diamond RD: Mechanisms of Resistance of Aspergillus fumugatus Conidia to Killing by Neutrophils In Vitro. *J. Infect. Dis.* 1985; 152(1): 33-42.

80. Galgiani JN: Inhibition of Different Phases of Coccidiodides immitis by Human Neutrophils or Hydrogen Peroxide. *J. Infect. Dis.* 1986:153(2): 21-22.

81. Pesanti EL: Pneumocystis Carinii: Oxygen Uptake, Antioxidant Enzymes, and Susceptibility to Oxygen-mediated Damage. *Infect. Immun.* 1984; 44(1): 7-11.

82. Brinkmann V, Kaufmann SH, Simon MM, et al: Role of Macrophages in Malaria: 02 Metabolite Production and Phagocytosis by Splenic Macrophages During Lethal Plasmodium berghei and Self-limiting Plasmodium yoelii Infection in Mice. *Infect. Immun.* 1984; 44(3): 743-6.

83. Murray HW: Cellular Resistance to Protozoal Infection. *Annu. Rev. Med.* 1986; 37: 61-9.

84. Paget TA, Fry M, Lloyd D: Effects of Inhibitors on the Oxygen Kinetics of Nippostrongylus brasiliensis. *Mol. Biochem. Parasitol.* 1987; 22(2-3): 125-33.

85. Ferrante A, Hill NL Abell TJ, et al: Role of Myeloperoxidase in the Killing of Naegleria fowleri by Lymphokine-altered Human Neutrophils. *Infect. Immun.* 1987; 55(5):1047-50.

86. Passwell JH, Shor R, Gazit E, et al: The Effects of Con A-induced Lymphokines from the T-lymphocyte Subpopulations on Human Monocyte Leishmaniacial Capacity and H_2O_2 Production. *Immun.* 1986; 59(2): 245-50.

87. Kazura JW, de-Brito P, Rabbege J, et al: Role of Granulocyte Oxygen Products in Damage of Schistosoma mansoni Eggs In Vitro. *J. Clin. Invest.* 1985; 75(4):1297-307.

88. Rothermel CD, Rubin BY, Jaffe EA, et al: Oxygen-independent Inhibition of Intracellular Chlamydia psittaci Growth by Human Monocytes and Interferon-gamma-activated Macrophages. *J. Immunol.* 1986; 137(2): 689-92.

89. Howells RE: The Modes of Action of Some Anti-protozoal Drugs. *Parasitology* 1985; 90(pt 4): 687-703.

90. Wirth JJ, Kierszenbaum F, Sonnenfeld G, et al:
    Enhancing Effects of Gamma Interferon on
    Phagocytic Cell Association with and Killing of
    Trypanosoma cruzi. *Infect. Immun.* 1985; 49(1): 61-6.

91. Ghadirian E, Somerfield SD, Kongshavn PA:
    Susceptibility of Entamoeba Histolytica to Oxidants.
    Infect. Immun. 1985; 51(1): 263-7.

92. Murray HW, Scavuzzo D, Jacobs JL, et al: In Vitro
    and In Vivo Activation of Human Mononuclear
    Phagocytes by Interferon-gamma. Studies with
    Normal and AIDS Monocytes. J. *Immunol.* 2987;
    138(8): 2457-62.

93. Podoplekina LE, Shutova NA, Fyodorov YuV:
    Influence of Several Chemical Reagents on
    Lymphocytic Choriomeningitis and Tacaribe Viruses.
    Virologie 1986; 37(1): 43-8.

94. Doroshow JH: Role of Hydrogen Peroxide and
    Hydroxyl Radical Formation in the Killing of Ehrlich
    Tumor Cells by Anticancer Quinones. *Proc. Natl.
    Acad. Sci. USA* 986; 83(12): 4514-8.

95. Zaizen Y, Nakagawara A, Ikeda K: Patterns of
    Destruction of Mouse Neuroblastoma Cells by
    Extracellular Hydrogen Peroxide Formed by
    6-hydroxydopamine and Ascorbate. J. *Cancer Res.
    Clin. Oncol.* 1986;111(2): 93-7.

96. Butler BD, and Hill BA: The Lungs as a Filter for
    Microbubbles. J. *Appl. Physiol. Respirat. Environ.
    Exercise Physiol.* 1979; 47(3): 537-543.

97. Shingu M, Yoshioka K, Nobunaga M, et al: Human
    Vascular Smooth are Susceptible to Hydrogen
    Peroxide. *Inflammation* 1985; 9(3): 309-320.

98. Didenko W: Possible Role of Lipid Peroxidation in the
    Pathogenesis of Arrhythmias in Myocardial Infarct.
    Biull. Eksp. Biol. Med. 1985; 99(6): 647-9.

99. Ward JF, Blakey WF, Joner El: Mammalian Cells are
    not Killed by DNA Single-strand Breaks Caused by
    Hydroxyl Radicals from Hydrogen Peroxide

Endothelial Cells Against Oxidant Damage. *Biochem. Biophys. Res. Commun.* 1985: 127(1): 270-6.

100. Pruitt Km, Tenovuo J, Mansson-Rahemtulla B, et al: Is Thiocyanate Peroxidation at Equilibrium In-Vivo? *Biochem. Biophys. Acta* 1986; 870(3): 385-91.

101. McFaul SJ: The Mechanism of Peroxidase-mediated Cytotoxicity. Comparison of Horseradish Peroxidase and Lactoperoxidase. *Proc. Soc. Exp. Biol. Med.* 1986; 183(2): 244-9.

102. Oya Y, Yamamoto K, Tonomura A: The Biological Activity of Hydrogen Peroxide. 1. Induction of Chromosome-type Aberrations Susceptible to Inhibition by Scavangers of Hydroxyl Radicals in Human Embryonic Fibroblasts. *Mutat. Res.* 1986; 172(3): 245-53.

103 Gutteridge JM and Wilkins S: Copper Salt-dependent Hydroxyl Radical Formation. Damage to proteins Acting as Antioxidants. *Biochim. Beefiest. Acta* 1983; 759(1-2): 38-41.

104. Tsan MF, Danis EH, Del Vecchio PJ, et al: Enhancement of Intra-cellular Gluthathione Protects Endothelial Cells Against Oxidant Damage. *Biochem. Beefiest. Res. Commun.* 1985: 127(1): 270-6.

105. Florence TM: The Degradation of Cytochrome C by Hydrogen Peroxide. *J. Inorg. Biochem.* 1985; 23(a): 132-41.

106. Del Prineipe D, Menichelli A, De-Mattis W, et al: Hydrogen Peroxide Has a Role in the Aggreation of Human Platelets. *FEBS-Lett.* 1985; 185(1): 142-6.

107. Agrawal P and Harper MJ: Studies on Peroxidase-catalyzed Formation of Progesterone. *Steroids* 1982; 40(5): 569-79.

108. Heikkila R and Cohen G: Inhibition of Biogenic Amine Uptake by Hydrogen Peroxide: A Mechanism for Toxic Effects of 6-Hydroxydopamine. *Science* 1971;172: 1257-58.

109. Zoschke DC and Staite ND: Suppression of Human

Lymphocyte Proliferation by Activated Neutrophils or H_2O_2: Surviving Cells have an Altered T Helper/T Suppressor Ratio and an Increased Resistance to Secondary Oxidant Exposure. *Clin. Immunol. Immunopathol.* 1987; 42(2):160-70.

110. Grisham MB, Perez VJ, Everse J: Neuromelanogenic and Cytotoxic Properties of Canine Brainstem Peroxidase. *J. Neurochem.* 1987; 48(3): 876-82.

111. Hell ML, Manson NH, Lower RR: Leukocyte-generated Hydrogen Peroxide Depression of Cardiac Sarcoplasmic Reticulum Calcium Transport. *Transplantation* 1983; 36(1): 117-9.

112. Verhoeven AJ, Mommersteeg ME, Akkerman JW: Balanced Contribution of Glycolyte and Adenylate Pool in Supply of Metabolic Energy.

113. Scott JA, Fischman AJ, Khaw BA, et al: Free Radical Mediated Membrane Depolarization in Renal and Cardiac Cells. *Biochim. Biophys. Acta* 1987; 899(1): 76-82.

114. Rubanyi GM and Vanhoutte PM: Oxygen-derived Free Radicals, Endothelium and Responsiveness of Vascular Smooth Muscle. *Am. J. Physiol.* 1986; 250 (5 pt 2): H815-821.

115. Eilin PJ, Strulowitz JA, Wolin MS, et al: Absence of a Role for Superoxide Anion, Hydrogen Peroxide and Hydroxyl Radical in Endothelium-mediated Relaxation of Rabbit Aorta. *Blood Vessels* 1985; 22(2): 65-73.

116. Wei EP, Christman CW, Kontos HA, et al: Effects of Oxygen Radicals on Cerebral Arterioles. *Am J Physiol* 1985; 248(2 pt 2): H157-62 Platelets. *J. Biol. Chem.* 1985; 260(5): 2621-4.

117. Kontos HA: Oxygen Radicals in Cerebral Vascular Injury. *Circ. Res.* 1985; 57(4): 508-16.

118. Burke TM and Wolin MS: Hydrogen Peroxide Elicits Pulmonary Artery Relaxation and Guanylate Cyclase Activation. *Am. J. Physiol.* 1987; 252(4 Pt 2): H721-32.

119. Hofmann C, Crettas M, Burns P, et al: Cellular Responses Elicited by Insulin Mimickers in Cells Lacking Detectable Plasma Membrane Insulin Receptors. J. Cell. Biochem. 1985; 27(4): 401-14.

120. Farr CF: (Unpublished Data) 1987.

121. Farber CM, Liebes LF, Kanganis DN, et al: Human B-Lymphocytes Show Greater Susceptibility to H_2O_2 Toxicity than T-Lymphocytes. J. Immunol. 1984;132(5): 2543-6.

122. Setty BN, Jurek E, Ganley C, et al: Effects of Hydrogen Peroxide on Vascular Arachidonic Acid Metabolism. Prostaglandins Leukotrienes Med. 1984; 24(2): 205-13.

Index

A

Acne, 48
Actinobacillus actinomy-cetemocomitans, 152
Acute and Chronic viral infections, 152
AIDS-Induced Brain Disease, 91
Air embolus, 33
Alka-Seltzer effect, 92
Allergic bronchitis, 42
Alzheimer's, 135, 151
American Cancer Society, 7
Angiology, 159, 160, 166
Ann. N.Y. Acad. of Science, 160
Arrhythmias, 151, 172
Arterial, 20
Arthritis, 6, 7, 16, 43, 47, 48, 71, 73, 75, 90, 95, 152
Ascorbic acid, 20, 81, 86, 167, 169
Aspergillus fumigatus, 153
Asthma, 42, 46, 137, 138, 151

B

B-cells, 42, 43
Bacillus cereus, 152, 170
Bacteria, 4, 6, 12, 13, 18, 19, 34, 38, 58, 63, 64, 68-71, 114, 152-154
Baylor University Medical Center, 23
Belle Glade, 69, 70
Bird Man of Alcatraz, 18, 19
Blastomyces, 153
Br. J. HematoL., 160

British Medical Journal, 33, 159

Bypass surgery, 24, 36, 45

C

Campylobacter jejuni, 152, 169

Can. J. Microbiol., 159, 169

Cancer, 3-7, 12, 23, 30, 31, 36, 37, 63-65, 69, 75-77, 79, 80, 83, 84, 97, 133, 134, 138, 160, 172

Cancer of the lung, 75

Candida, 19, 43, 47, 52, 85, 86, 88, 90, 101, 102, 152, 170

Candida albicans, 88, 152

Cardiac resuscitation, 25, 166

Cardioconversion, 151

Cardiovascular Disease, 3, 151

CAT scan, 79, 80

Catalase enzyme, 15, 67

Cerebral vascular accident, 110

Cerebral Vascular Disease, 151

Chelation therapy, 24, 41, 45, 78

Chelox therapy, 41

Chemotherapy, 31, 36, 63, 79, 80, 83

Chlamydia psittaci, 153, 171

Chronic fatigue syndrome, 43, 85, 86, 108

Chronic obstructive pulmonary disease, 46, 109, 151

Chronic pain syndromes (multiple etiologies), 152

Chronic polysystemic candidiasis, 47

Chronic Recurrent Ebstein-Barr Infection, 151

Chronic sinusitis, 42

Chronic unresponsive bacterial infection, 152

Circulation, 17, 25, 26, 33, 41, 43, 50, 78, 93, 160

Cleveland Clinic, 5

Clinical Science, 159

Cluster headaches, 152

Coccidioides, 153

G

Gingivitis, 19
Gott, Peter, 5, 6
Govoni, 34, 160
Grotz, Walter, 7, 95
Group B Streptococci, 152, 170

H

Haldone, J.S., 3
Hart, George, 26
HBO, 13, 24, 30
Health Freedom News, 159
Hepatic Dysfunction, 88
Herpes Simplex, 151
Herpes zoster, 109, 110, 151
Herxheimer reaction, 35, 89
High output heart failure, 25, 53
Histoplasma capsulatum, 152, 170
HIV infections, 152
Human Immunodeficiency Virus, 153
Human killer cells, 16
Hydrogen dioxide, 15
Hyperbaric oxygen, 3, 4, 12, 13, 16, 21, 23, 24, 26, 30,
      67, 93, 166
Hyperoxia, 23
Hypoglycemia, 84, 88, 110
Hypoxia, 25

I

Immune globulin fractions, 42
Immune Rebound Phenomenon, 52
In-Vitro, 160, 165
Influenza, 4, 41, 52, 108, 109, 151
Inotropic effect, 25

T

T-cells, 42
Tacaribe virus, 153
Temporal arteritis, 45, 46, 151
Tepanosoma cruzi, 153
Tex. Rep. Biol. & Med, 160
Thyroid, 20, 70
Toksikol, 161
Tomato Effect, 9
Toxoplasma gondii, 153
Treponema pallidum, 152, 169
Trichomonas vaginalis, 153
Tumor, 4, 30, 31, 79, 80, 154, 168, 172
Turnicliffe, 9

U

Ulcerative colitis, 33, 34, 55

V

Varicose veins, 75, 108
Vascular headaches, 152
Ventricular fibrillation, 25-28
Viruses, 19, 70, 114, 155, 154, 172
Vitamin C, 6, 20, 81, 82

Y

Yeast, 19, 47, 48, 85, 87, 89, 102, 121, 154